FOCUS ON THE FAMILY

SLEEP
IT DOES A FAMILY GOOD
how busy families can overcome sleep deprivation

DR. ARCHIBALD D. HART

Tyndale House Publishers, Inc.
Carol Stream, Illinois

A Focus on the Family book published by
Tyndale House Publishers, Inc., Carol Stream, Illinois 60188

Focus on the Family and the accompanying logo and design are federally registered trademarks
of Focus on the Family, Colorado Springs, CO 80995.

TYNDALE and Tyndale's quill logo are registered trademarks of Tyndale House Publishers, Inc.

All Scripture quotations, unless otherwise indicated, are taken from the *Holy Bible, New Interna-tional Version®*. NIV®. Copyright © 1973, 1978, 1984 by International Bible Society. Used by permission of Zondervan Publishing House. All rights reserved. Scripture marked (KJV) is taken from the *King James Version.*

The case examples presented in this book are fictional composites based on the author's clinical experience with hundreds of clients through the years. Any resemblance between these fictional characters and actual persons is coincidental.

The use of material from or references to various Web sites does not imply endorsement of those sites in their entirety.

Editor: Brandy Bruce
Cover design by Mark A. Lane II
Cover illustration copyright © by roccomontoya/iStockphoto. All rights reserved.

Library of Congress Cataloging-in-Publication Data
Hart, Archibald D.
Sleep, it does a family good : how busy families can overcome sleep deprivation / Archibald D. Hart. — 1st ed.
p. cm.
"A Focus on the Family book."
ISBN 978-1-58997-609-2
1. Sleep—Health aspects. 2. Families—Health and hygiene. I. Title.
RA786.H323 2010
613.7'9—dc22

2009044905

Printed in the United States of America
1 2 3 4 5 6 7 8 9 / 15 14 13 12 11 10

A Personal Note to My Clients—Past and Present

The personal stories I share in this book do not reflect any real person or persons. They are composites drawn from many cases as well as conversations I have had over the years in my seminars. Nevertheless, I owe you a note of gratitude for the trust you have bestowed on me in sharing your personal lives and the enormous wisdom I have derived from our conversations. I have tried hard to conceal any resemblance to actual cases, and I tell the stories in this book in narrative form only to make it more readable and my points more understandable. I love and respect so much all the clients I have seen over many years that I would never do anything to embarrass you or break the confidentiality you have entrusted to me.

Contents

PART 1:
UNDERSTANDING YOUR FAMILY'S NEED FOR SLEEP

PART 2:
DETERMINING YOUR FAMILY'S SLEEP PROBLEMS

PART 3:
OVERCOMING YOUR FAMILY'S SLEEP DEPRIVATION

Acknowledgments

No book is ever published that is not the product of many minds and hands, and this book is no exception. It is always humbling to be a part of the team that brings birth to a work like this, and a special joy to be a part of all that it takes. It is appropriate, therefore, that I pay tribute to all those who have assisted me in this project. I am profoundly indebted to each and every one of them.

First and foremost, I am indebted to my gorgeous and loving wife, Kathleen, who has always been a source of encouragement and inspiration to me. A pastor once described her as "Jesus in a dress"—and there couldn't be a more apt description of her than this. She was the one who many years ago alerted me to the importance of sleep and has led the way back to a healthier life for both of us.

Following closely are my three daughters, Catherine, Sharon, and Sylvia, who have all been a major source of inspiration in my life. Their gifts may vary, but their spirit of love and dedication to God's Kingdom is astounding. It has been my privilege to be a father to the three most beautiful girls in the world—beautiful in every sense of the word.

And then there are my grandchildren, Vincent, Alan, Nicole, Ashley, Robbie, and Daniel, as well as Matt and Mitch, who are all the greatest gifts and blessings God could give any grandparent. They are all that a grandparent could possibly want, and I am proud of every one of them. So proud, in fact, that I am dedicating this book to them.

And then last, but not least, I want to acknowledge the incredible help and support that the staff of Focus on the Family's publishing department has given me from the outset. Larry Weeden, director of book development, a friend for many years, stepped up to the plate when he heard I was writing a book on sleep and offered his support. Cami Heaps, author relations, picked up the ball and ran interference for me, guiding me through the maze of publishing. And then came the sensitive and remarkable insights and editing skills of Brandy Bruce who took over and shaped my flimsy initial manuscript into the sharp, readable (I hope) book that I believe it has become. In the background were other Focus staff members, such as Nancy Shane, Brock Eastman, and Shari Martin (product marketing). Thank you all for your dedication.

Introduction

Adam's birthday party Saturday? Check. Church on Sunday? Check. Presentation at work on Monday? Check. Dentist appointment Tuesday afternoon? Check. Change the oil in the car Wednesday afternoon? Check. Jane's soccer game Thursday? Check. Grocery shopping . . . I can fit that in on Friday, right? Check. Sleep? I wish!

Does any of this sound familiar to you? If so, you're not alone. If you were to take a good look at your family's schedule, sleep probably wouldn't even make the to-do list. It's a part of our lives, but not important enough to prioritize. But the truth is that it's alarming how little most people know about the life-ruining and mood-threatening consequences of not getting enough sleep. Couples don't realize that research has clearly identified bad sleeping habits as a major cause of marital distress. And our contemporary zeal for cutting back on sleep has consequences for our children as well.

The evidence, as I will show, is clear that most of us are not getting enough sleep, and this can be dangerous to the family. There is an indisputable connection between insomnia and both your physical and emotional health. How well you sleep can even affect how long you will live. And if you are a person of faith, healthy sleep habits have a lot to offer your spirituality. God has designed into us a need for sleep, as He has for all of nature. No person or creature is exempt.

But diagnosis without a remedy is never helpful. Just identifying your sleep issues isn't enough. The primary purpose of this book is to help you create healthier sleep attitudes and habits in your whole family. We can all sleep well again; we can all learn to fall asleep in a timely fashion and then stay asleep. It doesn't matter how long you have been in the grip of some insomniac monster; you can rebuild healthy sleep habits if you want to. If I didn't believe there was a solution to our struggle with sleep, I wouldn't bother to write this book. I've been there, done that. I resolved my struggle with sleep a long time ago, and it has made all the difference in my life. And it's precisely because I have conquered the beast of sleeplessness that I take this opportunity to share my conquest with you.

This book has three parts: In Part 1, I will lay a foundation of understanding about sleep. Understanding why and how we sleep is essential to remedying any sleep-related problem you or your family might suffer from. Why must we sleep? Why must we dream? What happens when we don't get enough sleep? We will explore the essentials of sleep so as to lay a foundation on which to build healthier sleep patterns.

In Part 2, I will help you diagnose your family's sleep problems and discover why sleep eludes you. Our ability to sleep soundly and adequately is not improving in modern times, but getting worse. The dominant influence of the Internet, including online social networks; cell phones, including texting; endless entertainment options; and much more gobble up our time. And since modern technologies are here to stay and in many ways serve to make life easier, it's imperative that all of us, grandparents included, understand how we can manage these potential sleep killers. Identifying the sleep-robbing habits and customs in both ourselves and our children, and knowing how to recognize the major sleep disorders, will open the door to effective solutions.

In Part 3, I will present ways to help improve your and your family's sleeping habits. I will lay out some key strategies for fixing your sleep problems, including when and how to use sleep aids, managing your family's "sleep bank," and protecting your marriage from the harm that comes from sleep-deprived irritability, intolerance, and sheer nastiness.

Feel free to read each part straight through or to skip around and find those areas that are of most interest to you. The fact is that sleep is vitally important for all of us, and my goal here is to help you move the priority of healthy sleep to the top of your and your family's agenda.

Because you've picked up this book, I know your desire is to improve the sleep habits of your family, and I applaud you for taking this first step. Being well informed about how you and your family can sleep better can only open the door to a healthier life together.

PART 1

UNDERSTANDING YOUR FAMILY'S NEED FOR SLEEP

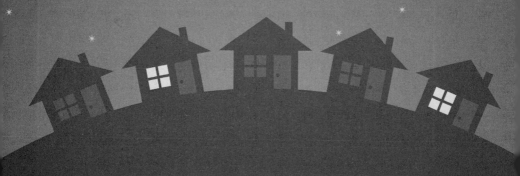

So Your Family Can't Sleep!

A flock of sheep that leisurely pass by one after one;
the sound of rain, and bees murmuring;
the fall of rivers, winds and seas, . . .
I've thought of all by turns, and still I lie Sleepless . . .

Even thus last night, and two nights more I lay,
And could not win thee, Sleep! By any stealth:
So do not let me wear tonight away:
Without Thee what is all the morning's wealth?
—WILLIAM WORDSWORTH, "TO SLEEP"

The call from Todd's school counselor came out of the blue. Fortunately Melissa, mother of 15-year-old Todd, was at home that morning. She wasn't feeling well and had taken the day off to rest.

"Mrs. Andrews, I am sorry to have to call you at home, but there is a problem with Todd's schoolwork that I need to talk to you about. When can we meet?"

Melissa had no idea that there was anything amiss. She called her husband, Jim, at work. "There's a problem with Todd at school, and the counselor wants to talk to us. . . . No, I have no idea what it's about; just tell me when you can be available so we can go see the counselor."

The counselor came right to the point. "I've received several reports from Todd's teachers that he falls asleep at his desk on a regular basis. They've tried chiding him, but it doesn't seem to be getting better. You need to look into the problem. Maybe he has a sleep disorder," the counselor suggested.

Jim and Melissa confronted Todd as soon as he came home from school. "It's no big deal. It's only happened a couple of times," he replied, dismissing the issue. But Melissa and Jim insisted on getting some help and came to my office for counseling.

At first, I met with only Jim and Melissa. I suggested they do a sleep assessment for Todd and gave them some tests to fill out, not unlike the assessment forms I'll present later. "And," I said, "please check Todd's cell phone records and see how often he uses his phone at night."

"Cell phone records?" Both seemed taken aback.

"Yes," I said, "cell phone records. Something must be keeping him awake until very late if you are sending him to bed at a reasonable hour. Trust me."

We soon found out that Todd had been text-messaging his friends until the early hours of the morning. He did it in the dark, under the covers, so his parents wouldn't know. It appeared that he was falling asleep around three o'clock most mornings, presumably from sheer exhaustion. He'd have kept going till sunrise otherwise. Todd did not have a sleep disorder—only lax family supervision! Welcome to the average American family.

A Sleepless Family

As a clinical psychologist, I also counsel couples with marital problems. I've seen a dramatic increase recently in marital conflicts that can be traced back to sleep problems. While we'll tackle the subject of marriage and sleep further in a later chapter, let's take a closer look at Melissa and Jim as an example. Aside from Todd's school problems, they had started having marital problems. Melissa was astute enough to link it to sleep deprivation as well. "We're becoming a sleepless family," she told me.

Melissa's main concern was with Jim. He had recently taken on a senior position at his company and was working longer and harder than ever before. It was not the hard work that was bothering her; she was confident he could handle that. But she had noticed subtle changes in his personality that had been upsetting her. He was becoming more irritable, less patient, and at times, even morose. Jim and Melissa had always prided themselves in having good communication skills as a couple, but lately Melissa just couldn't get a word through to him. What was most painful for Melissa was that their children had started to notice the change in their family atmosphere and were avoiding Jim because "he wasn't nice to be around anymore!"

As the three of us sat together in my office, Melissa said, "Jim isn't coming to bed as early as he did before. He seems restless and wants to stay up late. He keeps saying he's not ready for bed. And it's not that he's preoccupied with work or working on a project. It seems he just wants to veg out and watch TV or play on his computer. He calls it his 'downtime,' but it seems more like 'up time' to me."

Jim didn't deny any of her complaints. "Things have changed. Now that I'm the senior manager, I have more things to worry about. When I'm home, I need a break and some personal time."

With a few focused questions it became clear that Jim was also beginning to experience some health problems—problems that are often related to sleep difficulties. Most notable were the headaches that came on as soon as he got home from work. In a recent physical exam his doctor had noted that Jim was gaining weight, his cholesterol levels were high, his blood pressure was elevated, and there were signs he was pre-diabetic. Jim just shrugged off these concerns and said, "I'll worry about those things later."

Research has shown a link between poor sleep habits and sleep apnea, heart disease, high blood pressure, diabetes, and even strokes, so I knew we needed to explore further Jim's sleep patterns.[1] Sure enough, Jim admitted that he was now only sleeping about four or five hours a night, sometimes staying awake all night—or so it felt. I finally convinced him that he was living dangerously, and not only was his family life suffering, but his spiritual life was as well. He no longer took time to pray and was usually too tired to attend church with his family. "I'm just too busy for all that," was his excuse.

By this time, Melissa was also taking a closer look at their older daughter Amanda's sleeping habits. Amanda was a freshman away at college. Bright and always at the top of her class, she couldn't quite explain why her studies suddenly weren't going well. I provided a sleep-assessment questionnaire and determined quickly that Amanda was clearly not getting sufficient sleep to facilitate any effective learning. There were many distractions: She liked staying up late with her friends; she had joined a chorale group that practiced until late in the evening, and when she finally got back to her room, homework was waiting for her attention; her roommate also had bad sleeping habits; and so on. On top of all this, Amanda had fallen into the habit of spending hours on her laptop at night, chatting online with her friends.

Fortunately, Melissa and Jim took their therapy seriously, and while progress was slow, the marriage was saved and the kids eventually got on the road to right sleep. I can't say that every situation I've dealt with has always been that life transforming, but I can assure you that with determination and discipline, your family can change their sleep habits, and with that, change your life for the better.

My Passionate Embrace of Sleep

Of the many reasons why I chose to write this book, one stands out above all others: Bad sleeping habits in either children or parents can have a devastating effect on the spiritual, emotional, and physical health of the whole family.

Before I plunge too deeply into our understanding of sleep and sleep disorders, allow me to share some of my personal sleep journey with you. It was 28 years ago that I first became interested in sleep research and suspected I was sleep deprived. I had just become the dean of the graduate school of psychology at Fuller Theological Seminary, but I continued my research in the area of stress and stress-related disorders. Because I am somewhat of a driven person, and academia can be a "publish or perish" environment, continuing my research and writing was imperative.

Sleeping only about six hours a night in those days, I was struggling to get my writing done, felt a perpetual grogginess, and developed high blood pressure. I was preparing to publish the first edition of my book *The Hidden Link Between Adrenaline and Stress*, and had decided to include a chapter on sleep. Not much had been written about sleeplessness to that point. While there were those who were beginning to sound the alarm that we were losing our grip on sleep, by and large the idea was that sleeping too much could actually shorten your life, not prolong it. People were trying to find ways to stay awake, not get more sleep.

Up to that point in my life, therefore, my strategy was to try to get by with less sleep. My father only slept about six hours a night, and my brother, two years younger and a successful businessman, only slept for about four or five hours. We were pretty much a sleep-as-little-as-you-can clan.

My brother ran his own trucking business in South Africa and told me many times that the only way he could be successful in his business was to sleep as little as possible. Trucks had to work all night, and breakdowns were frequent. Customers expected on-time deliveries and accepted no excuses. So he became caffeine dependent, probably providing that industry with half its annual profits all by himself! Whereas he had chosen a business career, I eventually became a psychologist, went into academia, and immigrated to the USA.

My brother and I had always been very competitive. He boasted that he would be a millionaire before me. I responded by saying I would publish more books than he would. We both tried to eliminate sleep so we could pursue our dreams.

Then stark reality stepped in. My brother had his first heart attack. His doctor had warned him that he was working himself to death. He nearly died. I was struggling to write and research, but creativity seemed to elude me. I would go to my office to deal with all the hassles of running an academic program; then I'd go home and hit my typewriter. (This was before word processors!) I would normally get a chapter done before midnight, then crash into bed. I tossed and turned most of the night. And when I came back to that chapter the next day, it was all-too-often worthless.

So I began to explore some of the emerging research on sleeplessness. The message was clear: Lack of sleep produced more stress, not less. Sleeping less was a handicap, not a mark of superiority over other mortals. I learned that sleep isn't just a time to rest weary bodies, but it serves a whole constellation of functions, not the least of which is creative thinking. So I tried an experiment on myself. I reversed my strategy. Why not skip trying to write at night? I decided to try getting to bed early and then doing some writing the next morning, before going to the office.

Obviously, there was some trepidation here. I feared that taking more time to sleep would mean less time for my work. Surely, I thought, this would only make matters worse. But I went ahead and took the plunge. My secretary rearranged my appointments to start later in the morning after I had spent the first few hours reaping the benefits of a good night's sleep and then getting some writing done.

It only took a few days to convince me of the two principles I have followed ever since. First, getting to bed earlier, and as a consequence getting more sleep, works wonders for my brain. Second, creative tasks are best accomplished earlier in the day, rather than later. As I explain in my book *The Hidden Link Between Adrenaline and Stress*, your creativity is highest when your adrenaline arousal is at its lowest.[2] My fear that spending more time sleeping would mean reduced time to do my work, and hence lower my productivity, was not justified. In fact, as I slowly increased my sleep time, to my amazement my efficiency and productivity increased. The time I lost by adding more sleep time was more than compensated for by my being able to work and write more efficiently. I made far fewer mistakes. My ideas came more easily. I completed my tasks faster.

And I have been a sleep propagandist ever since. I teach it; I preach it. And now, as we will see, there is abundant research evidence to support my contention that the benefits of getting more sleep are more than compensated for by improved efficiency. I have proven over and over again that when I am well rested, I am at my best in every sense—even as a husband, as my wife will attest. This can be true for you as well. As we go through this book together, I'll help you determine the right amount of sleep for yourself and your family. So keep reading!

Sleep Is Essential to a Full Life

As I lay the foundation for understanding sleep, there is an important point I need to stress up front—and it's really a theological one. I cannot get away from the belief that God has designed sleep into us as a fundamental need, as fundamental as eating food and breathing air. In ancient times this need was more clearly understood. But in our modern times, the need for sleep is often misunderstood and even dismissed as unimportant by many, including some in the medical establishment.

One of the severest insomniac patients I have ever seen was a physician who abused his sleep patterns. He shared with me once that he believed sleep was some sort of evolutionary mistake; that we really don't need as much sleep as we think we need. Unfortunately, his sleep deprivation led to a severe addiction problem. To this day, I don't think he has resolved his addiction to self-prescribed drugs and alcohol.

Since it's so important in shaping our sleep attitudes, let me drive the "fundamental need" point home a little further. Sleep is not an evolutionary accident, as some would make out. God designed sleep to be an essential drive in nature. All nature sleeps. Even trees sleep in the winter months. Their sleep cycle is one year, unlike ours, which is one day. Some animals sleep all winter. Imagine what would happen if they all rebelled and refused to hibernate for the winter! Right now it's wintertime where I live, and my whole garden has gone to sleep! It's drab and brown—a literal eyesore. But I know that it will awaken in the spring and be beautiful once again.

Even though many millions of us are tired every day and know that we are not getting enough sleep, we turn a blind eye to it. Why is this? The answer is that, for the most part, we tend to associate sleeping long with laziness.

There's another reason why people avoid sleep, and it's one most of us can easily understand. Resting in bed while waiting to fall asleep often gives people time to think about things they'd rather forget. Sometimes the only time available for worry is when we lie down to sleep. A client recently shared this with me: "As long as I can run around and be as busy as a bee, nothing bothers me. But the moment I lie down to go to sleep, my mind becomes active and wants to revisit every moment of the day and find more for me to worry about. I hate going to bed. It's the worst time of my day!"

Although many questions about the role of sleep remain unanswered, scientific studies have shown that sleep contributes significantly to several important cognitive, emotional, and performance-related functions. We'll take a closer look at this throughout the book. Sleep is, in essence, the food the brain needs to survive, and not getting sufficient sleep is like starving your brain—it can be harmful, even life threatening. In short, sleep is essential to a full, rich, and satisfying life.

Some Sleep Problems Are Common— and Dangerous

The National Sleep Foundation (NSF) has conducted many polls over the past several decades exploring the incidence of sleep problems in adults, women, teenagers, and children. They report that about 70 million Americans suffer from some sort of sleep disorder. But that's only part of the problem. Many others suffer from some form of periodic sleep deprivation. These people have developed disruptive sleep or lifestyle habits that interfere with their normal sleep cycles.

Sleep deficits have been implicated in many major public catastrophes, including the oil spill of the Exxon Valdez and the destruction of the space shuttle Challenger. The nuclear accident at Chernobyl was also blamed on sleep deprivation, as were the near nuclear accidents at the Three Mile Island and Peach Bottom reactor sites.

Beyond these catastrophic consequences, the NSF polls have revealed that the cost of sleepiness to everyday humans is also astonishing. For example, each year there are more than 30,000 deaths from car accidents linked to sleepiness, and more than three million disabling injuries result from sleep-related accidents. Now I realize that I've taken quite a bit of space here to drive home the seriousness of our sleep problem. But I do so because it is important that we understand its seriousness.

A poll by the NSF in 2000 also estimated that an astounding 62 percent of American adults (basically, two out of every three of us) were not getting the amount and quality of sleep that their bodies and minds require. When repeated in 2005, the poll showed that this figure had risen to 75 percent. And by all accounts, it's still growing. According to the NSF, three out of every four American adults now have a sleep problem of one sort or another. The following figure gives us an idea of the percentages of people suffering from symptoms of insomnia.[3]

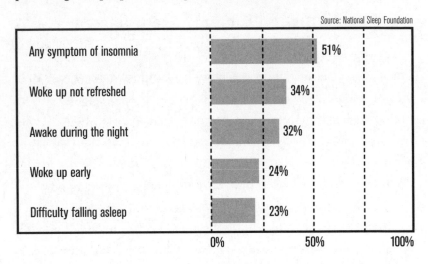

Source: National Sleep Foundation

Any symptom of insomnia	51%
Woke up not refreshed	34%
Awake during the night	32%
Woke up early	24%
Difficulty falling asleep	23%

0%   50%   100%

FIGURE 1: Percentage of Adults Who Suffer from Insomnia

Consequences of Sleep Deprivation

Let's take a closer look at the effect of sleep deprivation on the family. In a fascinating and informative segment on *60 Minutes* called "The Sleep Crisis" (March 30, 2004), Dan Rather reported that their review of sleep research showed that the lack of sleep was taking a heavy toll on American families. Children, toddlers, and even infants have the most to lose if they are sleep deprived. "Because we live in a 24/7 world, sleep is no longer a priority for the average American," he stated. And he's right. I would go a step further and say that not only is sleeping a low priority for many, but we have lost our respect for it. In other words, sleep has become an intrusive obstacle in our lives.

So what happens if a family doesn't get enough sleep? Our sleep loss can affect how we crouch, stoop, push or pull large objects, handle small objects, write with a pen, learn new things, remember old things, gain weight, walk up stairs . . . and the list goes on and on! As I go through an abbreviated list, note any you or your family might be suffering from.

Sleep deprived people:

- lose their ability to be joyful, lighthearted, and happy;
- tend to become irritable and negative;
- are at increased risk for accidents (a friend of mine crashed into the back of a garbage truck once, after a sleepless night);
- show a dramatic reduction in creativity and productivity;
- have memory problems;
- have disordered social relationships; and
- have a greater risk for divorce. (Sleeplessness aggravates our brain's anger center and disrupts marital relationships.)

On the physical side, even more serious health problems for family members are associated with sleep deprivation. A major study that epitomizes the gravity of our modern-day sleep deprivation reports that reduced sleep carries a greater mortality risk than smoking, high blood pressure, and heart disease.[4] Take a moment for that to sink in. Lack of sleep reduces your coping ability, so you become more stressed—with stress often comes elevated blood pressure, cholesterol, and so on. And stress is also a sleep disrupter, so it's a no-win situation.

According to the Institute of Medicine, the cumulative long-term effects of sleep loss and sleep disorders are associated with a wide range of serious health consequences, including a higher risk for:

hypertension (particularly connected to sleep apnea),

diabetes,

obesity,

depression,

heart attacks, and strokes.[5]

Further evidence that sleep deprivation is damaging to the family comes from what we pay for it. According to the U.S. National Commission on Sleep Disorders, almost 20 percent of all serious car crash injuries in the general population are associated with driver sleepiness, and that does not even take into account the sleepiness felt by those driving under the influence of alcohol. They also commissioned a study to determine the direct cost of accidents that result from sleep deprivation. The results were staggering. In the year studied, the cost of motor vehicle accidents in the U.S. that were attributed to sleepiness was more than $56 billion. And consider the fact that every crash victim was a member of a family somewhere.

Every parent knows that when small children don't get enough sleep, the whole family pays the price for their crankiness. This applies to Mom and Dad, too. When Dad insists on catching the late-night TV show and Mom can't put down her favorite novel until the early hours of the morning, they invariably get into an argument the next day. Missing out on sleep destabilizes the mood of the whole family. Show me a sleep-deprived family and I will show you a disorganized, unhappy family.

Even sleep-deprived babies can influence a family's well-being. In extreme cases, the crying and frustration of an exhausted baby can raise anger levels in parents that regrettably can lead to child abuse. It's well known that child sleeplessness can also lead to an increased risk of depression and anxiety in mothers, and a reciprocal loss of love feelings toward the child.[6] So you see, child sleeplessness affects not only children but the whole family system. I am sure that every parent reading this book has experienced (and remembers well) the profound effects of crying newborns—and that's only the beginning of the sleep challenge. (We'll offer more help on this important subject in chapter 9.)

Of course, those nights with a crying newborn don't last forever. But sleeplessness continues to plague children with learning disabilities, stress, and attention deficit or hyperactivity disorders when they get older. Sleep problems follow them into older childhood and the teen years with devastating effects on family life. This is perhaps the most compelling reason why sleep habits and sleep disorders should be prominently featured in the training of those involved in the health care of children, such as pediatricians, child psychologists, school counselors, and psychiatrists.[7] It's best to establish healthful sleep habits early.

"We Have Become a Nation of Insomniacs"

So says Mary Sykes Wylie, columnist for *Psychotherapy Networker*, a journal for mental health professionals.[8] "If a vast conspiracy were afoot to create an entire civilization of insomniacs," she says, "it would operate pretty much the way our society does now."

Insomnia. We either deny its existence in our lives or wear it as a badge of honor! For most, it's a dreaded word. But most of us experience it at one time or another. The nights spent staring at the ceiling counting minutes, or sheep, or whatever; desperately wanting to get some slumber time; worrying about how you will feel or perform the next day. The tossing and turning . . . waking up, then falling asleep, then waking up again. Finally, morning comes and you struggle to get out of bed, but a heavy cloud seems to follow you through the day. Your afternoons are spent in a daze. Basically, you're ready to fall asleep on the job at the slightest opportunity. And then there's the inevitable groping your way to the coffee machine or nearest "caffeine den" to get your java fix. Woe betides anyone in shouting range if the pot is empty or the shop closed.

What a grim life insomnia offers! And even though we all make choices every day that affect our ability or inability to sleep, there are other, more encompassing, reasons for exhaustion as well. Researchers blame cultural, sociological, and economic factors for turning what used to be transitory episodes of sleeplessness into a condition of chronic insomnia that now plagues the lives of many.

Types of Insomnia

Now let's look more specifically at the more common sleep disorders. Insomnia, the most common sleep disorder, can be grouped according to the cause, frequency, and duration of the problem, or how the sleep disturbance is experienced.

- *Primary insomnia* is when your difficulty in sleeping is *not* caused by another condition, such as an illness, or a drug, food, or drink. If you have the flu or a cold and you have difficulty sleeping because your nasal system makes it difficult for you to breathe, this is not primary insomnia.

- *Secondary insomnia* is a sleep disturbance that is caused by another problem such as illness, chronic pain, caffeine, or tobacco use. We all suffer periodically from bouts of secondary insomnia. It goes away when we treat the underlying condition.

- Difficulty falling asleep at bedtime
  - Termed "sleep-onset insomnia" (the sleep switch isn't working properly)
  - Defined as requiring more than half an hour, on average, to fall asleep

- Waking up and lying awake during the night
  - Termed "'sleep-maintenance insomnia"
  - Example: regularly lying awake during the night for a half hour or longer after having already slept for a while

- Waking up too early in the morning
  - Termed "sleep-terminal insomnia"
  - Often occurs in disorders such as depression and anxiety, or when you anticipate a heavy new day.

- Waking up tired because sleep is not restful

A Simple Sleep Test

How can you know if you are sleeping well? It's quite simple. Here are the signs of a well-rested body. See how many of them apply to you:

- You should have fallen asleep within half an hour of going to bed.
- If your sleep was disturbed, you should have been able to fall asleep again quickly.
- You should be waking up every morning at about the same time and feeling refreshed and alert.
- You should not be waking up wishing you could go back to sleep again.
- You should not have to use an alarm clock to wake up. (By all means set one up as a backup.)
- You should not be waking up with a headache or a feeling of fuzziness.
- While you might feel like taking a nap at noon, the feeling should quickly pass away.
- You should not feel sleepy at any other time of the day.
- You should be able to fall asleep again without difficulty the next evening.

If this does not describe your typical sleep habits, your sleep routine may be ready for a sleep makeover! However, you may also be suffering from an unrecognized sleep disorder. I will explore these with you later in the book, so that you can build healthier sleep routines for yourself and your family.

Most researchers agree that our society is now so chronically sleep deprived that even a small reduction in your normal sleep time can have serious consequences for the safety of yourself and others in your family. Fifty years ago, if you lost a few hours sleep a night for a few days, you could quickly recover. Today, you can't afford to lose even five minutes of your precious sleep time without a penalty. One researcher confirmed this by showing that even the small shift in our annual daylight savings time (DST) can have a major impact on car accident rates. Using data from two years of Canadian traffic accident records, he found that on the Monday following the shift to DST in the spring (when we lose an hour's sleep), there was an increase in the traffic accident rate of about 7 percent. In the fall (when we get an extra hour of sleep), there was a decrease in the accident rate of about the same magnitude.[9]

How Much Sleep Do We Need?

In 1960, a study by the American Cancer Society asked one million Americans how much sleep they were getting each night. It turns out that the median was 8 hours. Today the median time spent sleeping has fallen to 6.7 hours, and it's dropping by the month! This means that there has been a decrease of more than 15 percent in our sleep time, in less than my children's lifetime.

The 1995 report of the National Commission on Sleep Disorders recommended that the average person should get a minimum of 7.5 to 8 hours of sleep a night.[10] No recent studies have disputed this. Please note that this was the minimum sleep duration recommended for a healthy adult.

Now, with this clarification, we come to the million-dollar question: "How much sleep do we really need?" The answer is not all that straightforward. While we have general limits, the amount of sleep needed can vary from person to person, and also from circumstance to circumstance. So this means that we must discover for ourselves the most appropriate length of sleep needed.

For instance, someone going through a time of high stress may need more sleep, while someone on vacation, after having made up for his or her accumulated sleep loss, may then need less sleep than normal. Also, someone studying for an exam should intentionally get more sleep, as well as someone who is fighting an infectious disease. Generally I need 9 hours of bedtime. When I am stressed I go to 10. If I am traveling or doing a conference and feel energized, my sleep need may drop back to 8 hours. Then after I get home from a conference, it may lengthen to 9.5 or even 10, as my brain and body recover from the overloaded activity.

So how can you determine how much sleep you need? I'll provide a simple strategy for this, which can also be used to help your children personalize their ideal sleep period.

First, there's one important point to keep in mind. If you're aiming for 8 hours of sleep, remember that this means actual sleeping time. To achieve a minimum of 8 hours of sleep, you have to be in bed for longer than 8 hours. You need time to wind down and start the sleep process. It could take 15 minutes, or it could take 45 minutes. So if you can only afford to be in bed for 8 hours, you will not be getting 8 hours of actual sleep. You need to plan on adding an additional 20 or 30 minutes to your bedtime.

The strategy for determining how much sleep time you really need involves slowly adding incremental amounts of sleep, while observing the benefits. It has to be done in small increments, say 15 minutes, to allow your brain to adjust its sleep-time clock. Here's how to do it, for yourself and your family:

1. For the first week, add 15 minutes of sleep time to your normal sleep. You can do so by going to bed 15 minutes earlier, or by setting your alarm clock for 15 minutes later. Don't worry if you just lie there

awake. Stay in bed so that your brain gets the message. After one week, evaluate how the change affects you. At first, adding extra sleep time can have a rebound effect—it may make you feel more tired. This is because your brain is rebelling and asking for more, not less. At the end of the week, evaluate your level of tiredness upon awakening, energy, efficiency, alertness, mental acuity, reduced daytime tiredness, and your general feeling of well-being.

2. You may not feel much different the first week, but continue for the second week anyway, adding a second 15 minutes to your sleep—up front or in the morning. This now means an added half hour of sleep. Continue this for the second week, and evaluate its effects at the end. You should begin to feel the benefits, even if only slightly.

3. Now continue with the next 15 minutes and repeat the process. The plan is to do this until you have reached at least the nine-hour sleep mark. Now you will have a better idea of what amount of sleep your body and mind really need. If the benefits peaked at eight and a half hours, then stick with that for a while. If nine hours, then go with that and make the necessary lifestyle changes to support it.

It takes time for your brain to change its habits, so give it time to adjust after each change. Once you have found your most effective sleep duration, stick with it for at least the next three months so that it becomes an established habit.

Parents Need to Take Control

There is one closing point I feel I must make before I put this chapter to bed. (I couldn't resist the pun!) It is imperative that parents step up to the plate and take control of their family's sleeping habits. Our children are facing enormous increases in their general stimulation. They are forced to multitask in ways that undermine effective learning, and they generally have too much excitement in their lives.[11] Without disciplined supervision, sleep loss will take its toll on our precious offspring. Consider the fact that in 2008 the *Washington Post* reported that naptime was increasingly becoming "a luxury that 4-year-olds can no longer afford."[12] Many schools were eliminating naps from the kindergarten curriculum so that the recovered 45 minutes could be devoted to learning, oblivious to the neurological consequences.

The truth is that healthful sleep habits do not come about by chance; they must be taught. Animals have the advantage in that they are largely driven by instinct, and nature will see to it that they get the sleep they need. But humans are not instinct driven. We require discipline and training. Without careful tutoring here and, if I may say it, modeling by parents, our children will be the losers.

To make matters worse, many of the wonderful gadgets we have today are not always sleep friendly. And while things such as cell phones, computers, and even video games can hold positive benefits for families, without moderation, they can also serve as a detriment. A recent study has reported that the most common reason why teens are excessively sleepy during school time is that they spend a lot of time, often into the early hours of the morning, talking, text-messaging, or twittering friends![13] This study, as reported in *Time* magazine, concluded that "a good night's sleep is rapidly becoming more elusive for the average American." Please understand that I'm *not* saying we need to get rid of cell phones or other useful items. I *am* saying that we must use our time wisely, and that means valuing sleep enough to give it the time it deserves.

My point is this: The family that sleeps well, lives well.

Why Do We Sleep?

Sleep is the golden chain
That ties health and our bodies together.
—THOMAS DEKKER (1572–1632)

It is a common experience that a problem difficult
at night is resolved in the morning,
after the committee of sleep has worked on it.
—JOHN STEINBECK

It's quite remarkable that Thomas Dekker, in his quote above, makes a connection between sleep, health, and our bodies. These words, which could easily have come from the latest textbook on sleep, were actually written over four hundred years ago! Born in London, he became an author and playwright, even collaborating with Shakespeare. While he probably knew very little about the science of sleep, he knew a lot about life. Imprisoned three times for debt, once for seven years and twice for "recusancy" (not attending church), one can only surmise that he found value in sleep through those difficult times. His quote certainly reflects a profound appreciation for sleep and its value in keeping us healthy and sane.

It's clear from the many seminars I have taught that most people don't have any idea why we must sleep, or even that healthy sleep plays an important role in shaping a family's mental, physical, and spiritual health. By and large, they take sleep for granted without appreciating its profound value.

So, why do we have to sleep? No, this is not a silly question. If we are to motivate our children to change their sleeping habits and buck the modern cultural trend that seems to favor less, not more, sleep, then we need to know as much as we can about the topic of sleep.

We are up against a lot of resistance here. Magazine articles cite all sorts of "sleep-beaters" (including Nobel Prize winners) who brag about how much they have accomplished with so little sleep. When Margaret Thatcher was prime minister of England, she was lauded because she only slept four hours a night—as if her not sleeping much was what made her a great leader.

The truth is that many people believe a person can function perfectly well on just four or five hours of sleep. However, this is a myth that falls into the "wishful thinking" category. Legendary short sleepers, like President Bill Clinton, like to think that they have succeeded in life because they don't sleep a lot. And this might be true to an extent. If you work yourself to the bone day and night, you are bound to achieve some success. But at what price?

I can match any list of "little sleepers" with life-giants who had to sleep longer than most of us to achieve their greatness. Sir Winston Churchill, the great British prime minister who stood up to Hitler, for one, insisted on adding an afternoon sleep, not just a nap, to his sleep time. In his memoirs he insisted that in this afternoon sleep you should put your pajamas on! Carl Jung, a famous European psychologist, also insisted on having an afternoon sleep, not just a nap.

Many who claim to get by on little sleep also want to believe that their good health can be attributed to their less-than-normal sleep time. But they don't always acknowledge how tired they feel. Also, they often don't accurately report the extra sleep time they sneak in now and again, such as falling asleep in church or in front of the TV.

There may be, here and there, some who genuinely can get by on very little sleep and who seem to suffer no serious health consequences.

But they are few and far between—and don't live on my street. Being super-human is the exception, not the rule. As sleep expert Dr. Thomas Roth of the Henry Ford Sleep Disorders center in Detroit has said, "The percentage of the population who only need five hours of sleep per night, rounded to a whole number, is ZERO."[1]

I want to suggest that you set aside any preconceived prejudice against sleep you might have, and take an honest look at what the best of science is telling us as you work through this book.

What Does Sleep Do for Us?

From elephants down to the fruit fly, sleep is universal. Elephants can sleep standing up, but must lie down to dream. Crocodiles actually don't dream at all. Some animals must sleep 20 hours a day; others need only two or three. Some sleep with each half of their brain taking turns, in order to stay vigilant.

Sleep is not just helpful for survival; it's essential to life. For example, when deprived of dream sleep, rats can only survive for about five weeks. But if rats are deprived of all sleep, they only live for about one week. This is also how long it takes them to die from starvation—five days. In this case, food and sleep are equally vital for survival.

Sleep not only affects how long animals live; it is also one of the strongest drives in the lives of animals. Sleep drives an animal's life from start to finish just as much as hunger or thirst does. It is extraordinarily difficult for most animals to go without sleep for longer than 24 hours.

According to Dr. Matthew Walker, the director of the Sleep and Neuroimaging Lab at the University of California, Berkeley, the functions of sleep are so important to our survival that nature takes the risk of putting us to sleep at times, such as nighttime when it is dark and we are most at risk for being attacked, robbed, or even killed. While in today's world we are protected by homes that have locks on doors and burglar alarms, imagine what it must have been like in very early times when people slept in caves or crude shelters made of twigs. Everyone was at risk of wild animals attacking or greedy thieves robbing. So even if sleeping can be dangerous at times, our bodies are wired to understand that we must do it.

Sleep and Your Brain

While sleep is important to many bodily functions, there is no doubt that the major beneficiary of sleep is our brain. Did you know that not getting enough sleep can prevent the brain from getting an adequate supply of oxygen?[2] This is why many sleep experts advise us to sleep in well-ventilated rooms, so we can increase our oxygen intake.

But sleep's effects are not just physiological. Too little sleep leaves us drowsy and unable to concentrate. It also leads to impaired memory, impaired physical performance, and reduced ability to carry out even simple math calculations. If dream deprivation is prolonged, humans will eventually hallucinate in a matter of days. Some experts believe that sleep gives our neurons a break—literally a chance to shut down and repair themselves. Without sleep, neurons become so depleted of energy or polluted with by-products of normal cellular activities that they begin to malfunction. Sleep also may give the brain a chance to exercise important neuronal connections that might otherwise deteriorate from lack of activity.

Also, less than six hours of sleep a night ages the brain faster, and your appearance goes down the tube as well! After all, the idea of "beauty sleep" has been around for hundreds of years. If you want a free face-lift, try sleeping longer!

Other research has explored how much sleep deprivation impairs one's performance. It turns out that sleeping for six hours or less, for just one night, is enough to reduce your ability to function the next day.

The second night of insufficient sleep drops it further, and the third still further. Imagine what those who sleep six or fewer hours on a regular basis must be losing!

What Happens When We Sleep?

Sleep is by no means the mystery that it was a hundred years ago, when many believed it was just the first step to death, and it was only by the grace of God that you woke up the next morning.

What happens when we sleep? After about 15 to 30 minutes of relaxation, the prospective sleeper reaches a stage of semi-consciousness, which is being neither awake nor asleep. You may think you're still awake because you can hear noises, but you are in the early stages of sleep. After a few more minutes, the sleeper suddenly falls into unconsciousness. This final shift from drowsiness to unconsciousness only takes a second or two, but no one has ever been awake to observe how it happens in them! (The stages of sleep are described in the following sidebar.)

The transformations brought about by sleep are quite obvious to any observer. Breathing slows down. The eyeballs turn up and out; the fingers grow cold, but the toes warm. Blood pressure falls rapidly and is lowest about three hours after the onset of sleep. We change positions from 20 to 60 times during the night, mostly without knowing it, and for a few moments every 90 minutes or so, we may return to near semi-consciousness or even wakefulness for a brief while. Then slowly (unless something like the beast of an alarm clock disturbs the process), sleep becomes lighter. Consciousness flickers, fails, flickers again, and finally the light of wakefulness is lit. And if we have had an adequate amount of sleep, we are ready to engage a new day.

Figure 2 shows a typical night's sleep and its various stages. Take a good look at it. You will notice that we sleep in 90-minute cycles—give or take a few minutes—and pass through each of the stages at differing speeds. After reaching the dream stage of sleep, you may wake up briefly or return to a lighter stage of sleep. This is when you turn over or adjust your sleeping position. Normally you can't remember doing this, but sometimes, especially if you're stressed, you could wake up fully and

---

The Five Stages of Sleep

Sleep comes in five distinct but closely interconnected stages:
- Stage 1: A drowsy, relaxed state where you are somewhere between waking and sleeping. It's the early stage you enter when you put your head on the pillow. Your respiration slows, muscles relax, and heart rate slows down. Most people who are awakened from this stage will report that they were "starting to drift off," but were really not yet asleep.
- Stage 2: A deeper but still light stage of sleep. Insomniacs are more likely to perceive stage 2 sleep as still being awake, but might be asleep and not realize it.
- Stages 3 and 4: The deeper stages of sleep. The brain starts to produce very slow waves as seen on an EEG. Here you reach the lowest levels of physiological activity during the 24-hour day.
- REM sleep (Rapid Eye Movement) is the deepest stage of sleep and is where we do most of our dreaming. It is very different from the earlier sleep stages that are quiet and referred to as NREM, or non-dream sleep. REM sleep is also described as a "waking brain in a paralyzed body." The body is paralyzed but the brain is working very hard.

then find it difficult to get back to sleep again. This is called a "sleep disruption," and many suffer from it regularly. Cumulatively, it could become a sleep disorder.

However, let me clarify that our natural sleep architecture takes us back to wakefulness or semi-wakefulness (stages 1 or 2) every one and a half hours or so, so waking up periodically is normal—provided you can fall back asleep again quickly. We sometimes wake and don't know it, especially if we have slipped back to stages 2 or 3. But waking up several times a night is quite normal, and if you are well rested, it has no consequences. It happens more often as you get older. People who are sleep deprived pass out for long periods, so sleeping through the night without waking may actually indicate sleep deprivation, especially if your total sleep duration is short to begin with.

Also, you will notice in the diagram that the duration of the dream stage gets longer as the night progresses. In other words, most of your dream sleep comes in the last cycle or two of your sleep, which is why a longer sleep period is more beneficial.

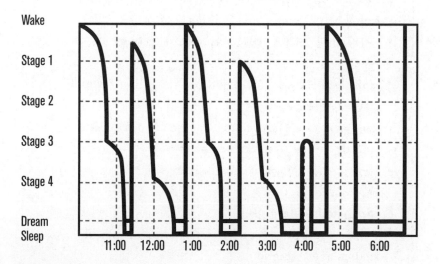

FIGURE 2: The Sleep Cycle

Notice that there are distinct cycles of sleep, going from light sleep to dream sleep. In this example there are five cycles. At one and a half hours per cycle, in total this includes about seven and a half hours of sleep and falls short on at least one cycle. So if you want to have a proper sleep, as opposed to just a nap, you have to commit yourself to between five and six cycles of sleep—my preference being the latter. Also, the next time you wake up naturally during the night, pay attention to the time that elapsed between going to bed and your waking. It will most likely be a multiple of around one and a half hours.

Functions of Sleep

Now let's look at the functions that sleep provides. Each of the stages mentioned previously have their own functions, and they play together like a well-tuned orchestra. Here is what each stage provides:

Stage 1:
- The mind and body are prepared for entry into sleep. It is the onset of a deep, relaxing state. Adrenaline and awareness drop slowly.
- Melatonin level also rises to facilitate sleep onset.

Stage 2:
- Semi-sleep occurs as awareness continues to drop and drowsiness sets in.
- This relaxed state helps restore energy. Glands like the adrenals are able to rest and rejuvenate.
- This stage also serves to help the body's muscles to rejuvenate.

Stages 3 and 4 (deep sleep):
- In these stages there is a release of growth hormone in children and young adults.

• Many of the body's cells also show increased production and reduced breakdown of proteins during deep sleep. Since proteins are the building blocks needed for cell growth and for repair of damage from factors like stress and ultraviolet rays, deep sleep rejuvenates us.

• If we are deprived of deep sleep, the brain will recover or "make up" deep sleep first before it will settle back into the other stages. Furthermore, loss of deep sleep produces the greatest impairment during daytime functioning compared to the loss of other stages of sleep.

REM sleep (or dream sleep):

• Here the brain processes information, like problems and new learning, and grows new connections accordingly.

• It synthesizes information learned through the waking hours.

• It saves newly learned information into long-term memory.

• And it facilitates forgetting (removal of short-term memory), a function often overlooked.

The Brain's Sleep/Wake System

There is an important connection between being asleep and awake. Humans are rhythmic. Our bodily functions are predictably controlled across the 24-hour day. Believe it or not, your brain has a complex time-keeping system. The most basic of our behavioral cycles is the sleep/wake cycle. Sleep serves as an "anchor" in the 24-hour day, around which our other bodily rhythms—hormonal, physiological, neurological, and behavioral—are synchronized. So in reality, our life revolves around our sleep cycle, not our wake time. Wakefulness is just a bonus! Here is a summary of our sleep/wake patterns:

• The Wake system promotes alertness during the day.
• The Sleep system promotes sleepiness at night.
• The Wake system is dominant for about 14 to 16 hours of a day, while the Sleep system is dominant for the remaining hours.
• The longer the Wake system is "on" during the day, the greater is the drive for nocturnal (nighttime) sleep and the better we sleep.

But not only is there a time-keeping function in the brain that keeps us on track for sleeping and waking, there is also a sleep "On/Off switch." Sleep comes and goes under the control of this switch deep inside the brain.

One of the interesting aspects of our brain's sleep/wake mechanism is how the moment we fall asleep occurs. One moment we are awake, and the next we are asleep. We don't take the final step into sleep slowly. We can't foretell when it will flip or flop. It happens so suddenly we cannot force or stop it!

The sleep switch is triggered in the brain by a chemical called hypocretin, which is the controller of wakefulness and sleep. When you have lots of it, you are awake, and when you have little of it, you fall asleep. Our brain does what hypocretin tells it to do; it's sort of the "master of the house," so to speak. Discovered only as recently as 1998, this chemical is now believed to be the boss over the whole sleep/wake cycle. For instance, if you don't get enough nighttime sleep, then your daytime sleepiness is due to a lack of this chemical. This is how the brain tells you that you're not getting enough sleep!

So, what's this got to do with you and me? Simply this: You have to cooperate with these systems if you're going to be a healthy sleeper. Difficulty falling asleep or waking up frequently could be due to too much hypocretin. Being unable to wake up is the reverse. To improve the efficiency of the sleep flip/flop switch, a number of exercises have been explored and found to be effective. The bottom line is that all stress has to be reduced if you are going to have enough hypocretin to keep your sleep switch healthy. Stress reduction, then, is key to a healthy sleep switch, as well as other strategies I will recommend later.

Nocturnal Versus Napping

Some years ago, my youngest daughter and her husband moved to Germany where my son-in-law's company was under contract with the air force. My wife and I took advantage of their three-year stay there and visited them as often as we could. They lived near a U.S. air force base out in the countryside. But we were most disappointed the first time we went shopping in the local village.

It was early afternoon, and I craved some good, old-fashioned German bread. But when we got to the bakery, it was closed. I checked the sign in the window, and it clearly stated that the bakery would not open again until after 3 PM. Closed from noon till three? I wondered how the shop could make any money with hours like those. But I soon found that there were signs saying the same thing in the windows of the grocery store, the knickknack store, and every other store in the little town. I was frustrated and confused, but all we could do was go back to my daughter's home and take a long nap ourselves. Welcome to sanity!

The fact is that in addition to the brain's clock telling us when to sleep and when to wake, there is also a drive toward an early afternoon mini-sleep that is universal in humans and animals. Yes, that early afternoon call to sleepiness is your brain's doing.

When sleeping, the temperature of the body starts to decline and is at its lowest in your deep sleep. Then it starts to rise again before waking. However, while the body's temperature is normal all through the morning hours, in the early afternoon it takes a minor plunge, and with it comes some drowsiness. Many cultures, through the ages, have taken advantage of this afternoon sleepiness and have developed siestas or napping practices. There's clearly a biological underpinning for the body's need for rest halfway through the day—something many of us try to ignore these days.

Six Ways to Restore Your Body's Clock

Disruptions to your brain's internal clock, such as when you do night-shift work or suffer from jetlag or daylight savings time changes, can interfere with your sleep patterns. Here are some strategies for resetting this clock and restoring the circadian rhythm of your body:

1. Go to bed at the same time every night. (Your brain's clock loves regularity.)
2. Get out of bed at the same time every morning.
3. Expose yourself to lots of daylight as early as possible. (It resets the clock.)
4. Darken your home environment one hour before bedtime. (Starts your melatonin.)
5. If you have to stay up late one night, get to bed earlier the next night. (Helps cancel your sleep debt.)
6. If you know your sleep will be deprived ahead of time, such as when traveling, try sleeping some extra time ahead.

Be patient if you can't sleep after your body clock has been disrupted. If you keep regular sleep times, your brain will eventually correct itself.

Figure 3 shows how our sleep drive fluctuates through a typical day. The night or nocturnal sleep has the greater drive. Since the Industrial Revolution, most modern countries have ignored the nap drive, and in many ways, we pay the penalty for this neglect.

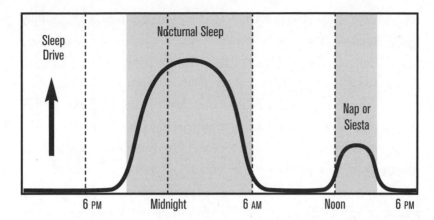

FIGURE 3: Nocturnal Sleep Pattern

But before I go any further, let me clarify a very important point because there is some confusion in the use of different terms. A nap is usually understood to be a short period of rest. It is not the same as sleep, unless it lasts for a complete sleep cycle and goes through all the sleep stages, including the dream stage. In other words, if you nap for one and a half hours, you are really sleeping, not just napping, and this counts toward your required sleep needs for the day.

Many of the cultures that embrace siestas are not just napping, but actually sleeping. And there is a difference. A short nap's benefit comes more from its value in helping us rest and lower our adrenaline (stress) levels during the day. I can nap for 20 minutes between delivering lectures and feel quite refreshed. It helps rejuvenate our stress systems and is, therefore, extremely helpful. But it really doesn't do much for the brain. We need proper sleep for that.

Given our drivenness to succeed at everything we do and our tendency to equate time with money, it is not surprising that we often view napping either as wasteful and self-indulgent, or as a sign of mental or physical weakness. And if these misperceptions control our lives, we pay for it in reduced levels of happiness and increased stress.

Research has found that napping is not only healthful and mentally beneficial; it can also make a vast difference in our vigor and reduce our late-afternoon lethargy.[3] About one-third of the population naps at least once a week—though many keep quiet about it. In fact, since naps often help to lower adrenaline, they may even foster better sleep. And while the elderly may nap more because they have the time for it, many others have discovered a wonderful secret: They function better and are more productive after they've had a nap.

Strong evidence for the value of napping also comes from a study in France.[4] This is interesting to me since the French already enjoy a 35-hour workweek and a minimum of five weeks of annual vacation. Wow! Who could ever really be stressed with such a work schedule? But it appears that one in three people in France suffers from a sleeping problem. To deal with the consequences of sleep disorders (work absenteeism, high rates of work errors, traffic accidents, low energy and concentration), the government investigated the role that naps can play in solving their sleeplessness problems. So they introduced the idea of letting workers nap at work. They set aside 15 minutes at lunchtime for a nap and discovered that workers' moods improved, worker relationships got better, absenteeism dropped, and workers felt less tired. And all from a midday 15-minute nap! They also found that the nap should not be longer than 20 minutes, and the sleep should be light.

Taking a regular daily nap also has one other benefit not commonly known: It can actually improve memory. This has colossal benefits for students of all ages, because improved memory means improved learning. What is also remarkable is that this benefit doesn't require a long sleep to achieve this. Studies have proved that sleep lasting 90 minutes really does build up the memory big time. But naps as short as 12 minutes can also provide a memory boost. Moms and dads need to remember this when it comes to our children's sleeping habits.

Now I realize that many readers cannot take a nap during the workweek, even if they wanted to. A busy bus driver cannot pull over and tell her passengers to wait while she takes a nap! A schoolteacher can't ask his students to excuse him while he takes a 15-minute nap. But what I do want to encourage here is for you to understand the value of napping and make the time, whenever you can, to embrace a nap. Even a five-minute nap, taken while waiting for an appointment or on the bus ride home from work, can lower your adrenaline significantly. It pays to be a little creative here.

So, why not put down this book right now and take a five-minute nap before proceeding? Your mind will be most thankful.

Why Do We Have to Dream?

Behold, this dreamer cometh.
—Genesis 37:19 (KJV)

*When I think my bed will comfort me
and my couch will ease my complaint,
even then you frighten me with dreams.*
—Job 7:13–14

If trying to understand why we have to sleep is challenging, trying to understand why we have to dream is even more so, but extremely important. Insomnia isn't just about a loss of sleep; it's also about a loss of dream sleep. In the last chapter, we looked briefly at dream sleep (REM) and non-dream sleep (NREM). Now we'll go a bit further in understanding the differences between those two. The truth is that non-dream and dream sleep go together. You need the one to get the other.

But the relationship between dream and non-dream sleep is a little more complicated. We may sleep for a long time but not get enough dream sleep. It's also possible to get too much dream sleep. Many commonplace medications, such as antidepressants, and substances like alcohol and caffeine may interfere with our dreaming, not just our sleep.

Non-dream sleep occurs in the earlier stages of sleep from stages 1 to 4 and is important for the restoration of the physical body. If you do heavy manual labor, you need more non-dream sleep. Dream sleep, on the other hand, is the deepest stage and is important for the consolidation of memory and learning, as well as for sorting and storing information in the brain. So if you do mental work, you need plenty of dream sleep. In fact, for people whose jobs include much critical thinking and brainstorming, insufficient dream sleep can cause them to wake up with headaches, apathy, poor judgment, increased sensitivity to pain, and a decrease in alertness.

About 25 percent of our sleep should be of the dream type, and the remainder should be non-dream. The lighter, non-dream sleep is important to dream sleep because it's only after a certain amount of non-dream sleep that you can pass into your dream sleep.

Protecting Your Dream Sleep

When we first go to sleep, we are in non-dream sleep. Then, after about every 80 or 90 minutes, we pass into dream sleep and stay there for a few minutes. After dreaming for a while, we return to a lighter stage of sleep or even wake up. It's important to not force yourself into full wakefulness during these periods of light, non-dream sleeping. Don't get out of bed unless it's essential, such as having to go to the bathroom. Eating a snack or watching TV is not a good idea, as it's going to move you to full wakefulness. Getting up usually opens up your adrenal valve and makes it more difficult to get back to a deep sleep again.

If you wake up after dreaming, try just lying in bed and relaxing. If your dream was bothersome, keep a notepad nearby and jot down what it is that's bothering you—in the dark, of course. This makes it easier for you to fall asleep again, because writing down what bothers you is like saving it to an "external drive," to use a computer analogy. My theory is that it tells the brain it's not important and you don't need to try to remember it. This helps in letting you drift back into a deep sleep again.

Dreams Fascinate

Throughout history, dreams have been a source of fascination. I imagine that in olden days people would sit around the fire on a cold winter's night and recount their dreams, embellishing them like fishermen's stories so that they became tales of intrigue. Or they might have told each other their dreams so that they could interpret them in ways that made for interesting conversation. It was a form of entertainment, and it certainly fostered a rich imaginative ability.

Furthermore, I believe sharing dream stories was probably a great source of comfort and provided, unknowingly perhaps, psychotherapy. No psychotherapists were needed in those days! Therapy was built into everyday life. And, no doubt, this is why dreams played a major role in telling life stories in early literature, such as in Shakespeare's plays.

In earlier times, dreams served two major functions in storytelling: to *provoke guilt* for past deeds and to *foretell events* to come. People worried a lot about the future because life was so uncertain. Many of Shakespeare's characters compare dreams with waking reality, often noting that things that seem real in dreams take on a reality of their own. People were never really sure about what was real and what was unreal in a dream.

But our concern here is with the role that dreaming (notice that I *don't* say "dreams") plays in shaping the mental health of your family. To understand the importance of dreaming, we need to know *how* and *why* dreams are generated.

Must We Remember Our Dreams?

A very common concern many have about dreams is whether or not they should be remembered. Most sleep experts agree that the meaning of most of your dreams is of no consequence. Dreams are just the random activity of your brain. However, some people are bothered by their inability to remember their dreams, and therefore fear they may not dream.

Emily is typical of many I have met in therapy or seminars. I had just delivered a lecture on sleep during one of my seminars and had made reference to our need to dream. Emily, a lovely woman of Chinese descent, had asked a few pointed questions during my presentation on dreaming, so I knew that she was troubled by the topic. It was no surprise when she approached me during the break and said, "Dr. Hart, I never dream. Honestly, I can never in all my life remember ever having had any dream." And then she broke into tears.

She was quite upset and went on to share how the topic of dreaming had been frustrating for her. For years she had been bothered about never recalling any dreams. She assumed that it was because she never dreamed, but here I was, insisting that we all dream. She had never shared her anxiety about not dreaming with anyone else. It seemed embarrassing for her. She'd never even told her parents about her lack of dreams. When she was young and anyone asked about her dreams, she would make up something.

To make matters more difficult, she told me, Chinese culture places a great emphasis on dreams and what they mean. Because she never seemed to dream, she believed there was something wrong with her.

I asked her about her sleep in general. She went to bed at a regular time. She had no depression and was not taking any medication that could be suppressing her dreams. She didn't drink alcohol. She consumed very little caffeine and generally got a good night's sleep. She wished she could get more sleep, but who doesn't?

So I gave her a quick homily about the unimportance of remembering your dreams. I want to repeat what I said to her here for the benefit of any readers who might also be troubled about the same issue. Here are the main points to remember about your dreams:

- Everybody dreams; the brain demands it. The question of whether you dream is not determined by what you remember. Most of us recall only a small percentage of our dreams.

- People who claim that they never dream, when taken to a sleep lab and their sleep patterns recorded, discover that they do, in fact, dream. They produce the identical dream brain waves as those who remember their dreams.

- Even if you're a good "rememberer of dreams," you still can't recall 90 percent of them. The reason is that while we dream, several times through the night (typically about six dream sessions), each subsequent dream cycle erases the memory of previous dreams. Dreams are generally not important to the brain, so it erases them. Dreams are sort of "short-term memory material." And it's in our dreaming stage that short-term memory is converted to long-term memory and stored. This is why we usually can only remember the last dream of the night. Or if an earlier dream was really scary or significant, the brain might just decide to move it into long-term memory. And then it might be difficult to forget.

- A high percentage of the population cannot recall their dreams. When pressed, Emily, the student mentioned earlier, admitted to me that she vaguely remembered having had some dreams. But it was all very indistinct in her memory, to the point where she wasn't sure it had really happened. I reassured her that there was nothing wrong and her anxiety was pointless. And if she really wanted to solve the problem, she could have a sleep recording done at a sleep lab that should settle the issue for her once and for all.

So don't worry if you can't remember your dreams. It's not important, and it's not a sign that anything is wrong with your sleep architecture. Just remember this: *That* we dream is important, not *what* we dream.

What Do People Generally Dream About?

Do people around the world differ in their dreams? This question has fascinated researchers for years. In the 1940s, a well-known psychologist named Dr. Calvin S. Hall started collecting dream stories from all around the world. He collected more than 50 thousand dreams and published a book about their contents.[1] A quick review of how common many types of dreams are might help dispel any anxiety you have about your dreams or the dreams any of your family may have shared with you. This is what Dr. Hall found:

Emotions
The most common emotion experienced in dreams was anxiety. Negative emotions are more common than positive emotions, and some ethnic groups showed an abnormally high rate of aggressive dreams. The U.S. ranks the highest among industrialized nations for aggression in dreams, with 50 percent of U.S. males reporting aggression in dreams compared to only 32 percent, say for Dutch men.

Gender Differences
In men's dreams, 70 percent of the characters are other men, while a female's dreams contain an equal number of men and women.

Sexual Content
Here we have a surprise. Unexpectedly, sexual content was not as prevalent in the dreams studied as was expected. Sexual dreams showed up no

more than 10 percent of the time, though they were more prevalent in teens.

Recurring Dreams

While most dreams usually occur just once, many reported recurring dreams. Sometimes they spring out of conflict, but not always. In my early thirties, I had a recurring dream about being in a small airplane with a pilot who has a heart attack and dies. I would struggle to take control of the airplane and panic because we might crash. Then I would wake up in a sweat and fear going to sleep again, in case the dream repeated itself. I believe that this dream started after I saw a movie with this theme as a child.

Years later, I took flying lessons, and from the day I went solo, the dreams stopped. I've never had that dream again.

Other Common Themes

The more common themes in dreams seem to be: situations relating to school, past work experiences, being chased, sexual experiences, falling, flying like a bird (this is my wife's favorite dream), being late, being partially naked in public, failing an examination, or having a car accident. Some dreams are in color; others are not.

Common themes are found across many cultures because they reflect common life experiences. We are likely to dream about things we fear or desire. I developed a hernia earlier in my life from lifting a heavy weight. I did not have it repaired right away, and even today I occasionally dream that my hernia has returned. Such dreams are natural and don't have any hidden or mysterious messages. They are just reminders of things that happened to us in the past and that we might fear could happen again. Many dreams are also simply re-experiencing past events. I often travel in my dreams to places in the world I have been to before. Even bad dreams have no hidden significance; they are merely expressions of our normal fears and worries.

The Functions of Dreams

What, then, does dreaming offer? Two decades ago, Dr. Rosalind Cartwright summarized what had been discovered about dreaming in the following renowned summary:

> The brain doesn't turn off when we go to sleep; it just switches channels. Dreams offer the three R's and in times of stress a fourth R. . . . They allow us to Review, Revise, and Rehearse the program of ourselves. And when life is tough, as in depression, they also provide a mechanism for Repair.[2]

It is not just in times of stress that dreams offer repair. This repair work happens every time we dream. Also, I would add a fifth R. Dreams help Restore the brain to full functionality in readiness for the next day's activities and demands.

Not only do dreams carry out the five R's, but they also help us to be creative. This is why your creative abilities rely heavily on dream time. I experienced the power of dream's creativity a year ago while designing a new biofeedback instrument. I wanted to upgrade an instrument I had developed years ago, and adapt it so it could be used for stress management on a laptop computer.

I worked for several weeks on the project, mastering one little step at a time. There were probably 30 problems to be solved or electronic modifications to be made. And then I had to rewrite the computer program that ran the whole gizmo. Each step of the project would require a whole new approach. I would struggle for a few days, drawing diagrams or writing sub-routines. Then after having teased out all the problems of each step, I found myself dreaming about the project and waking up in the morning with a solution staring me in the face. But it wasn't the dream that presented the solution to me. Rather, my brain had dreamed on it, and when I awoke, it gave me the answer I had been looking for.

This has happened to me many times. In fact, the night before I wrote this chapter, I went to bed with a house-repair problem on my mind. I didn't have a clue as to how I was going to repair the problem. I woke up briefly at 3 AM, and there was the solution, staring me in the face. It's as if I had "seeded" my brain with the problem before falling asleep, then my brain dreamt on it, and when it was ready with a solution, it woke me up and presented it to me. I have had this happen to me time and again; as I am sure many readers have as well.

Dreaming and Learning

Another important function of dreaming is how it facilitates learning. What is it in our dreaming that helps us learn? Mainly, dream sleep helps the brain do two things: It helps it rehearse what has been learned, and then it consolidates what we have learned. When we learn something new, the learning is not complete until we go to sleep. It is then that the "connections" practiced during, say, repeatedly playing a piano piece, are made more permanent in the brain. This is such a crucial insight that every parent and schoolteacher need to know about it. However, many teachers I have spoken to have never heard about the role in learning that sleep and dreaming have.

Some fascinating studies are currently (2009) underway at the Sleep and Neuroimaging Lab at the University of California, Berkeley. After studying more than four hundred subjects, researchers found that if you sleep after learning a new task, when you come back the next day you perform the task even better than you did when learning it. Just "sleeping on it" improves performance 30 percent or more. For example, subjects who learned a complex task in the morning and were tested in the evening (before they could get any sleep), did not do as well as subjects who were tested the next day, after a good night's sleep.[3] While sleeping, the brain continues to practice whatever it has just learned. This is one of the reasons why it's not a good idea for college kids to cram their learning into the early hours of the morning at the expense of sleep. A good night's sleep, after spending some time learning, is essential to retaining what you have learned.

Improving Your Dream Sleep

Now we come to the practical application of what we have learned thus far. How can we improve our dream sleep? Since I will provide more detailed and practical help for improving general sleep later, all I want to do here is point out a few critical factors that can affect and possibly improve your dreaming:

- The easiest way to improve dream sleep is to avoid any substance that might interfere with your dreaming, including the following:
  - alcohol and nicotine (they both repress dream sleep)
  - caffeine (it suppresses all sleep)
  - some drugs used for high blood pressure (don't take more than you need)
  - some antidepressants (the older types of antidepressants especially, as some of them inhibit REM sleep)
- Dream sleep can also be facilitated by ensuring enough time for your total sleep.
- Some emotional and mental health problems can seriously interfere with your dream sleep. In clinical depression, for instance, you might spend more time in the deep stage 4 sleep,

and thus get less dream sleep. Anxiety disorders tend to reduce dream sleep as well. Turning and tossing all night keeps you in a lighter stage of sleep. Post-traumatic stress sufferers, such as soldiers returning from war or people who have been in a serious car accident, can also experience reduced dream sleep. Also, their dreams can become nightmares. People suffering from fibromyalgia or other neurological pain disorders can also experience dream-sleep interruptions. A number of medical conditions can also disrupt dream sleep, including asthma, chest pains, bronchitis, bladder problems, prostate problems, allergies, emphysema, diabetes, hyperthyroidism, and headaches. Fortunately the sleep problem goes away when the medical condition is resolved.

- Lastly, nightmares and night terrors are never compatible with good dream sleep. So if you suffer from either of these things, you're most likely not getting the dream sleep you need.

Dealing with Bad Dreams

Aside from nightmares and sleep terrors (which I will deal with in a later chapter), many people suffer periodically from what are described simply as bad dreams—dreams that may not be nightmares, but nevertheless are unpleasant and can rob one of a peaceful sleep.

I've had spells of bad dreams. When we first married, my wife had a series of miscarriages. Every time my wife became pregnant, she miscarried after a month or two, and we didn't know why. Finally, we sought out a specialist, and he put my wife on a special hormone supplement. My wife was soon pregnant again, and everything with this pregnancy seemed to be normal.

So far, so good. But I started to have bad dreams. In my dreams, my wife continued to have miscarriages. The dreams were so bothersome that I dreaded going to bed at night. But the more I tried to avoid the dream, the greater was the likelihood that I would have it. Sadly, when our child was nearly at full term, she died in the womb from hydrocephalus, a condition where fluid builds up around the brain. My wife and I were devastated. But thanks be to God, my wife's next pregnancy was perfect, as were the two that followed. We now have three beautiful, intelligent daughters, all with doctorates, who are the joy of our lives.

On a related note, it's quite common for pregnant women to have severe and vivid bad dreams about things going wrong with their pregnancy. There are no hidden messages in such dreams. In fact, it would be unusual not to have such dreams, because pregnancy always carries some risk. Internet blogs are full of dream stories about pregnancies gone wrong. One I saw recently told of a pregnant mother who one night dreamed that her unborn baby developed an infection and died. The next night she dreamed she went and had an abortion, something she would never choose to do. The following night, in her dream, someone came and removed her baby and took it away. She would wake up after such dreams in a cold sweat.

One way to reduce such nightmares is to intentionally talk out your fears with someone you can trust, or even journal them. The more courageous you are in facing these fears, the less likely you are to have the nightmares.

While some bad dreams may be serious enough to warrant seeing a sleep specialist, you can usually deal with them yourself. Before closing this chapter on why we dream, let me leave you with a very useful strategy for countering repeated bad dreams. It was the strategy I used early in our marriage when I was plagued with unpleasant dreams, and it has been used successfully by many of my clients.

Many cultures practice something called "dream incubation," where one tries to create certain dreams intentionally. The use of this strategy can, at times, help eliminate bad dreams. This is how it works: If you don't want to have a certain bad dream, then intentionally tell yourself, when you are going to sleep, that you wouldn't mind having the dream. Better still, write out a brief description of the dream before you go to bed; then read it aloud and tell yourself it's okay if you have this dream.

Why does this work to block a bad dream? It's the paradoxical nature of wanting to have a dream, even if it's unpleasant, that helps block the dream. If you try to "incubate" a dream, the chances are high that you will actually suppress such a dream—this is true for all dreams, good and bad. Try it yourself the next time you go to bed. Think of a dream you would like to have. Then see if you have it. As far as we can tell, it just doesn't happen most of the time.

If you find it too scary to test a bad dream, then try the strategy by trying to create a good dream first and see if it suppresses that dream. Then try creating a bad dream and see what happens. It's possible that welcoming or confronting bad dreams head-on actually lowers your anxiety about having them. It's as if you are telling your brain that there is nothing to be afraid of, often resulting in a peaceful night's sleep.

The same principles can be applied to children who have bad dreams. But first you must deal with whatever may be scaring a child in his or her waking moments. Some of the things that our children are being exposed to on a daily basis may be triggering bad dreams and nightmares. Topping the list is the newer and very scary trend we see in TV shows, as well as commercials. Violent crashes, with car and body parts being thrown into the air, are common in movies and TV shows.

While older children can become immune to such violence after repeated exposure, young children go through a period when it can trigger bad dreams, since they cannot always tell what is and isn't reality. Halloween time can be especially threatening to many young children. Corpses rising off tables, blood spewing out everywhere, and monsters jumping out of nowhere are not conducive to a child's peaceful sleep.

Parents need to carefully monitor what their children see on TV and at the movies. Don't leave your TV on when you are not around. Set up whatever TV protection device you can to make sure your children are exposed only to age-appropriate scenes.

Can you remember your childhood nightmares? Mine were mostly about monsters hiding under my bed, or my falling from the top of a high building. It just so happens that when I was a child, I would climb on our roof quite often, mainly to retrieve kites or balls. And my bad dreams, even today, often have me falling off high places. I don't recall it, but my parents tell me that I once tried to make a parachute out of an umbrella. After all, it was shaped like a parachute. I climbed up the drainpipe onto the roof over the kitchen, opened the parachute (umbrella), clung tightly to the handle, shouted "Geronimo!" and ended up in the hospital with a broken arm.

For quite some time afterward, my mother says, I would wake up screaming at night after a bad dream. She never talked about it with me, fearing that talking about it would trigger the nightmares. But if she had talked about it with me, I believe my dreams would have subsided. While very young children, say under five or six years of age, may just need a lot of loving care and assurance when they go to bed after a bad experience, older children need to learn how to interpret such bad experiences and see their bad dreams as normal experiences. So before your child goes to bed, have him tell you about any bad dreams he is having. Let him draw a picture of whatever the creature was that was hiding under the bed. Let him give him a name— preferably a funny one. Then let your child crumble the paper and throw it far away, to show that it is nothing to fear, just an imaginary thing.

But it is important that, as much as possible, you do not let your children experience any fearful event. Don't send them into the dark to fetch something, especially if you know they are scared. My father did that several times when there was a power failure. For a while, as a child,

I became afraid of the dark. Also, never scoff at your children's fears if something does scare them. Their feelings are very real. Your children need to know they can come to you with anything bothering them and never be laughed at. Your caring responses and reactions to your child's fears can help him or her rest in the security of your love and protection.

PART 2

DETERMINING YOUR FAMILY'S SLEEP PROBLEMS

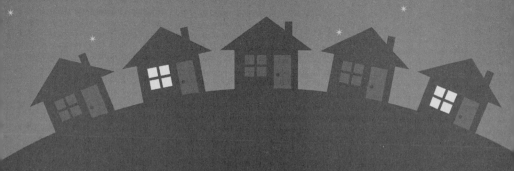

Why Can't Your Family Sleep?

O sleep, O gentle sleep, nature's soft nurse,
How have I frighted thee,
that thou no more wilt weigh my eyelids down
And steep my senses in forgetfulness?
—WILLIAM SHAKESPEARE, *HENRY IV*

It's late in the evening and you still have e-mails needing replies. There are also a couple of bills to pay online, and, oh yes, there's that latest episode of your favorite reality show you TiVo'd earlier in the evening, awaiting your attention. By the time you finally crawl into bed, it's well past midnight. But this isn't unusual for you; it's your regular nighttime routine.

Now, though you are in bed, your mind is still active and you can't switch it off. Something about that last e-mail just before turning off the computer is on your mind. You ponder the thought that you might just get up again and reply to that e-mail in case you forget it in the morning. You play the "Should I? Shouldn't I?" game. A part of your brain reminds you that if you don't get to sleep soon, that darn alarm clock will scream extra loud at you when 6 AM arrives.

So you decide not to get up. You'll deal with it in the morning. But will you remember? You ask yourself, *Should I get up and make a note of it?* Have you noticed that when you have to remember something, your mind keeps waking you up to remind you? So you lie there, eyes wide open, waiting . . . wishing . . . hoping . . . that "gentle sleep, nature's soft nurse" would come "and steep your senses in forgetfulness." Shakespeare must have known something about insomnia to write such an evocative verse! When that alarm finally does wake you, you want nothing more than to just stay where you are.

But that's not the end of it. Drowsiness and fatigue follow you all through the next day. You catch yourself nodding off at your desk or workbench. You can't remember what it was your boss told you to do. In fact, you always struggle to remember things in the morning. It's as if your memory system has been turned off. You promise yourself that you're going to get to bed earlier tonight, but there is little willpower to resist staying up late and cramming in as much as you can during your waking hours. Sleep seems like such an intrusive thing, a waste of good time and a spoiler of happiness. Why can't you find a way to get rid of it? You fantasize about inventing a vaccine that takes away the need for sleep. You're sure you could make a fortune!

Sleep Killers

There are many reasons why you or a family member might not be getting a good night's sleep. Some are mundane. As a teenager, my younger brother, who shared the same bedroom with me, would often come home late at night, interrupting my sleep. It was the source of a lot of conflict. He insisted on turning on the light when he entered so he could get changed; this would inevitably wake me up and we'd end up in a shouting match. Of course, getting mad only made it more difficult for me to get back to sleep. One night I unscrewed the lightbulb in our bedroom so he couldn't turn the light on. And while I was a very happy boy waiting for my brother to come home (and losing quite a bit of sleep because of it), it only created more of a ruckus. Finally, I just resigned myself to the intrusion and figured out a way to cover my eyes with a part of my blanket. What I would have given for a pair of eye covers and earplugs!

While there can be many reasons why we can't get enough sleep, there are four overlooked sleep killers that need highlighting here:

Sleep Killer #1: Stress

Stress is by far the most important cause of disrupted sleep facing us today. The accelerated pace of life, coupled with the reduced time we set aside for recovery, drives many of our sleep problems. In short, stress has never been as intense and pervasive as it is today. Stress can destroy our sleep potential as certainly as a hole in a ship will sink it.

Stress and insomnia are closely linked in the following ways:

- Stress releases powerful hormones that disrupt sleep—notably cortisol. In an emergency your body cannot be allowed to sleep. There is work to be done or battles to be fought. This is not the time to sleep!
- Prolonged stress (called "chronic stress") creates a state of perpetual emergency. There is no interruption to the adrenal system, and consequently there is a continuous interruption to sleep. Also, sleep problems can persist long after the stress has passed away.
- The lack of sleep reduces our stress-coping ability, creating a vicious cycle. With reduced coping ability, even minor stressors can become major sleep killers.
- Eventually, sleeping less becomes a habit—one that is difficult to break.

It's here that we can see a possible reason for a connection between the incidence of heart disease and poor sleeping habits. The excessive production of stress hormones like adrenaline is associated with increased risk of cardiac death. And since elevated adrenaline also inhibits sleep, there must inevitably be a connection between the two. According to a study conducted by researchers at London's Westminster University, healthy sleep can lower the stress hormone cortisol. In excess, cortisol, a cousin of adrenaline, is responsible for some depression and anxiety disorders.[1] It's not clear which comes first in this chicken-and-egg situation. Is it the lowered adrenaline and cortisol that helps us sleep better and protects our health, or is it the extra sleep that lowers the adrenaline and cortisol? It doesn't really matter which comes first, because we need to safeguard both.

The heart-disease sufferers I have studied over the years, including my brother, father, and uncle, all confirmed my suspicion: They had poor sleeping habits, as I did earlier in my life. It goes with being a Type A personality. They don't sleep enough; they sleep lightly; they can't get to sleep easily; or if they do fall asleep, they wake up early and then can't get back to sleep again. Their minds are active, and they are too excited or fearful most of the time. Their thoughts won't give the adrenal system any peace. Instead of sleeping, they use the nighttime to plan how they will finish projects, clinch a sale, think up new challenges, fight their battles in fantasy, or worry about the next day. I know. I'm as guilty as anyone!

Not surprisingly, many of these high-risk individuals paradoxically find it quite easy to sleep during the daytime—or on a couch in front of the television set. But the moment they go to bed, their sleep need vanishes. This phenomenon is worthy of some careful research!

Sleep Killer #2: Anxiety and Worry

Anxiety and worry are also significant sleep destroyers. As Charlotte Brontë once observed, "A ruffled mind makes a restless pillow." So some attention also needs to be given to strategies for dealing with anxiety and worry. This topic requires more attention than we can deal with here. You can consult my book *The Anxiety Cure*[2] for specific help. Also, I will address the topic of worry in a later chapter when I present some strategies for sleeping better.

Sleep Killer #3: Caffeine and Caffeine-Related Drinks

You might be squirming at the thought of having to give up that cup of coffee you enjoy so much, but bear with me. Eighty-five percent of the U.S. population drinks caffeine-laced beverages.[3] Caffeine is so well integrated into our culture that many people don't even think of it as a drug. However, according to Dr. Roland Griffiths of Johns Hopkins School of Medicine, "When you get down to it, caffeine is a drug and it needs to be accorded the same respect as a drug."[4]

Furthermore, Dr. Griffiths reports that people aged 65 and over drink more coffee than the rest of the population. Three hundred million cups of coffee, most laced with caffeine, are consumed in the United States each day, making it the second most commonly traded commodity in the world.

It is particularly important that parents manage their children's caffeine intake, as this could develop into a lifelong addiction. Caffeine is common in many sodas, and because of its addictive properties, parents could be creating lifetime addicts by neglecting to regulate its consumption in their home.

Unfortunately, the coffee industry is making a strong push to present the good side of coffee. They remind us that coffee is an antioxidant. When you compare men who drink coffee with those who don't, it appears that coffee can reduce the risk of type 2 diabetes by 50 percent. In the elderly, drinking coffee can improve memory and energy (after all, caffeine is a stimulant). But most of this research intentionally avoids comparing caffeinated versus decaffeinated coffee.

It's the coffee, not the caffeine, that is the antioxidant, yet news reports trying to show coffee's benefits seldom share that important point.

The debate here parallels that of the liquor industry trying to show that red wine can prevent heart disease, but then failing to warn drinkers to not consume it more than two or three times a week. The bottom line here is that just because a substance has some good qualities, does not mean there are no dangers associated with its other qualities.

So what about the bad side of caffeine? First, because it's a stimulant it can be misused. It can mislead people into thinking they don't need more sleep when in reality they are only being kept awake by the caffeine. Also, it's powerfully addicting. Caffeine is a mild diuretic and increases secretion of fluids from the body, which can lead to confusion and dizziness, as well as causing the elderly to fall, according to an Oxford University health journal.[5] Withdrawal symptoms, such as headaches, are common. Caffeine intoxication is now a recognized disorder in the *Diagnostic and Statistical Manual of Mental Disorders,* published by the American Psychiatric Association.

But my greatest concern here is caffeine's effect on sleep architecture. It's a major cause of insomnia and anxiety disorders. It keeps us awake, which is why we drink it. Many see coffee (its caffeine) as a solution to daytime sleepiness. In reality, while it might wake you up temporarily, it only adds to the sleep problems now plaguing our society.

Also, caffeine undermines the effect of tranquilizers you might be taking. So if you suffer from anxiety and need to take a tranquilizer, you should stop consuming caffeine.

The overall issue here is that we should consume caffeine moderately. Control when you drink your favorite caffeine beverage. Remember that it has a half-life of 7.5 hours. This means that 7.5 hours after you have consumed caffeine of any kind, including the now-popular power or energy drinks, half of the caffeine is still in your system. After another 7.5 hours, a quarter is still in your system. The effects of caffeine, therefore, hang around for a lot longer than most people realize. The nearer to bedtime you consume it, the greater its disruptive influence on your sleep will be.

Caffeine is a two-edged sword—it both overcomes and causes our sleeplessness. It's no wonder that almost every sleep expert I've encountered cautions against over-using caffeine in any form. The increased consumption of caffeine during the college years only leads to insomnia—a habit that can stay with these college students for the rest of their lives.

Michael's story is typical. "I like to think," he says, "that I lead a normal life. I graduated from a prestigious university; I have a full-time job; I own my own home; I have a beautiful wife and two adorable kids; and I'm, in general, an all-around, middle-class, Christian American success story. Except for one thing: I am an addict."

Michael doesn't drink alcohol. Nor does he do drugs or even smoke cigarettes, but he learned his addiction during his college years. And when he talks about his addiction, he often gets a strange look and a response like, "Who isn't addicted to that?" He is referring, of course, to his addiction to caffeine. Whether it's coffee or Mountain Dew, he drinks a lot of it every day. It was the late-night cramming for exams and college activities that ate into his sleep time and got him hooked on caffeine. He just couldn't function without it, and as with all addictions, he had to keep increasing his intake just to get a fix. His sleep patterns were chaotic. By the time he sought help, he had become quite ashamed of his addiction and was concealing from his wife just how much he consumed. She was the one who discovered just how serious his addiction had become.

He will be the first to tell you that quitting his caffeine addiction has not been easy. Even after a couple of years of therapy, he still has a mammoth struggle to just keep his intake at a moderate level. He takes some consolation in his now being open about his addiction and trying to warn others, especially college-age kids, of just how serious an addiction this can become. It can be as challenging as alcohol to quit—perhaps more so, since society generally doesn't even see it as a problem.

To illustrate the effect of caffeine on sleep duration, consider Figure 4. Note the drop in total sleep and in dream sleep after consuming caffeine at different levels, and the drastic drop after 300 mg when hardly any dreaming occurs.

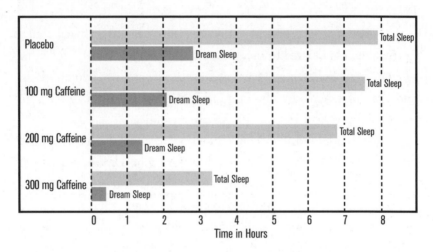

FIGURE 4: The Effects of Caffeine on Sleep Duration

If you are a caffeine lover, doctors recommend you only drink two to three cups of coffee per day and stay away from all energy drinks since they are high in caffeine. And if you're one of those people who feels like you can't function without coffee or other caffeine-based stimulants, then it's time to make a change in your life.

Although giving up caffeine altogether is the best option, if you are already addicted to or dependent on it, there are ways of making it work in your favor rather than against you. For some caffeine addicts, drinking a cup of coffee about an hour before going to bed mellows out their

---

COUNT YOUR CAFFEINE

While I generally advise my patients to avoid major caffeine drinks, most experts recommend limiting your caffeine to less than about 200 mg. Older people, say over 70, who cannot metabolize caffeine well, and anyone with a chronic insomnia problem should avoid all caffeine. We should all avoid caffeine after 3 PM. To estimate your TOTAL DAILY caffeine intake, examine the table below and count your caffeine intake as conscientiously as you count your food calories.

Decaffeinated coffee (8 oz.)	Less than 10 mg
Regular coffee (8 oz.)	Around 100 mg
Hot cocoa (8 oz.)	Less than 10 mg
Tea: instant and brewed (8 oz.)	30 to 40 mg
Red Bull (8.2 oz.)	80 mg
Mountain Dew (8 oz.)	55 mg
Cola (12 oz.)	About 40–55 mg
Sprite, 7-UP	Zero
Hershey Bar (1.5 oz.)	About 10 mg
Excedrin (2 tablets)	130 mg
No Doz: Regular Strength (1 tablet)	100 mg

FIGURE 5: Count Your Caffeine

system, thus helping them get to sleep. But this only works for someone whose body has become dependent on caffeine.

If all else fails and you suspect that caffeine is still causing problems for you when trying to sleep, you could try over-the-counter sleeping pills or even something as simple as warm milk. (We'll explore the good and bad news about sleeping pills later.) Warm milk has lactic acid in it that releases a chemical when warmed, and this often triggers a natural sleep cycle. A baby will likely go to sleep right after having a bottle of warm milk, and the same principle applies to adults as well.

One caution however: If you stop using caffeine suddenly, you are likely to experience withdrawal symptoms, notably headaches. And they can be very severe. A Johns Hopkins Bayview Medical Center report on caffeine dependence clearly states that the higher the caffeine intake, the more likely a patient is to suffer from severe withdrawal symptoms when denied the ingredient.[6] If you plan on stopping or lowering your caffeine intake, you may want to talk to your doctor first.

The symptoms start within 24 hours of the last serving of caffeine, peak within two days, and then start to subside. However, they can last longer than a week. While many experts recommend moderation (not necessarily abstinence) in caffeine ingestion, as in many addictions, some will not be able to limit their intake. If this is you, I recommend giving it up altogether.

Sleep Killer #4: Depression

A recent study (published in the journal *Sleep*) reported that in a longitudinal study where young adults were monitored over a long period of time, insomnia and depression were often seen together.[7] For a long time we have believed that insomnia might be causing depression, not the other way around. But it now appears that it's the depression that is

---

Caffeine Withdrawal

A report from Johns Hopkins University, published a few years ago (based on the findings of more than 60 studies on caffeine withdrawal), gave five withdrawal symptoms to look for:
- headaches (the most common symptom)
- fatigue (over-stimulation depletes energy)
- mood changes (including depression)
- inability to concentrate
- flu-like symptoms

causing the insomnia. Depression and depressive symptoms are the largest and most consistent risk factors for insomnia. And with the epidemic of depression now occurring in our teenagers, this connection must be heeded.

I have already written extensively on the topic of depression, so I will not repeat myself here.[8] But keep in mind that if you or any member of your family has any signs of depression, bouts of insomnia are likely.

Lifestyle Habits That Disrupt Sleep

Some years ago, a friend who worked in downtown Los Angeles shared with me some of the struggles he was having in his life. He was a senior executive in a world-renowned company and his job was very demanding. It required a lot of international travel, and this meant getting up very early. Living in our area, it also meant a commute into Los Angeles that often added several hours of driving to and from his workplace every day. Needless to say, he had to get up early and often arrived home late. The net result was that his sleeping habits were chaotic. When we sat down and drew up a schedule of his average day's activities, he was barely getting four or five hours of consistent sleep.

Then it happened. Walking to his car in the parking basement of his company's high-rise, he started to feel an excruciating pain in his chest. Yes, a heart attack. He was fortunate to have a colleague walking with him, who promptly got him to a hospital.

After his triple bypass, we sat down together and talked about how his lifestyle—working at some distance from where he lived, taking on work responsibilities that were not his own, always accepting some increased responsibility in his company just to prove he was exceptional at what he did, and above all, never getting a normal night's sleep—was killing him.

After some serious talking, he took control of his lifestyle. First, he requested that he be moved to a less demanding position in the company. Yes, his salary would be lowered, but he was earning a good salary to begin with. Second, he talked it over with his family, and they decided to move to a location where he could commute to work by train. This would get him home earlier and allow him to relax on his way to and from work. Third, I convinced him to take a proper lunch break and to take a half-hour break every mid-morning, at which time he would go to a park near his office. He still does this today, 10 years later.

Many lifestyle habits can also disrupt your family's sleep. And all it takes to come up with the changes you need to make to get back on the sleep train is a little common-sense review of your lifestyle. Here we will assess a few of the more important lifestyle challenges and point you to some habits that need changing:

- Lifestyle Stressors: Without realizing it, you may be doing things during the day or night that can work against getting a good night's sleep. These include drinking alcohol or caffeinated beverages in the afternoon or evening, exercising close to bedtime, following an irregular morning and nighttime schedule, and working or doing other mentally intense activities right before or after getting into bed.

- Shift Work: If you are among the 17 percent of employees in the United States who are shift workers, sleep may be particularly elusive. Shift work forces you to try to sleep when activities around you—and your own "biological rhythms"—signal you to be awake.

- Jetlag: Still another sleep stealer is jetlag. This inability to sleep is caused when you travel across several time zones and your biological rhythms get "out of sync."

- Physical Factors: Disorders that cause involuntary limb movements during sleep, such as Restless Legs Syndrome, break up the normal sleep pattern and are also likely to make sleep less refreshing and result in daytime sleepiness. For women, pregnancy and hormonal shifts, including those that cause premenstrual syndrome (PMS) or menopause and its accompanying hot flashes, can also intrude on sleep.
- Medications: In addition, certain medications, such as decongestants, steroids, and some medicines for high blood pressure, asthma, or depression, can cause sleeping difficulties as a side effect.

Analyzing Your Sleep Disruptions

We all have differing and unique patterns of sleep disruption—somewhat like having differing fingerprints. Identifying your unique sleep disruptions can be useful in designing a better lifestyle that fosters sleep. While I touch on several of these disruptions in other parts of the book, particularly in the last section, where I offer remedial help for sleep problems, let's briefly examine the more important ones here, so you can determine which ones might be hindering your family's sleep routine.

- Noise Interferences: Noise is extremely disruptive to sleep. You need to be assertive and deal with outside sources of noise. Your neighbor's dogs, teenagers, and even your own pets need to be reined in so that you can get a good night's sleep. Suggestions on how to do this will come later. For now make a note of them.
- Other Environmental Interferences: A distracting sleep environment (for example, a room that's too hot or cold, too much traffic noise from a nearby freeway, a room not dark enough, etc.) can become an obstacle to sound sleep. Also, the comfort and

size of your bed and the habits of your partner can affect your sleep.

- Overactive Children: Night interruptions from children or other family members who cannot sleep can also disrupt your sleep. You may have to exercise some discipline and ingenuity to get kids to bed on time—and to keep them in bed.
- Pain: A common disrupter that many leave unattended is pain. Sudden, severe pain can make you bolt upright from a sound sleep. But even milder pain can cause "micro-arousals." These are periods when your pain breaks through, and while it doesn't necessarily wake you, it bumps you back into a lighter sleep stage, robbing you of deep sleep.

Please note that it's not just the intensity of pain that can upset your sleep. Intensity can vary widely; it's often the variableness of pain that is more disrupting because your body cannot adapt to it. If you have a steady pain that lasts many months and is predictable, your brain may be able to get used to it. Pain can throw your whole life out of whack if it's untreated, so don't hesitate to get treatment for it.

Just Because Your Family Doesn't Feel Tired Doesn't Mean They Don't Have a Problem

This speaks to one of the main points I want to make in this chapter: Even though you (or your children for that matter) may not feel tired, this doesn't mean you don't have a problem. Self-perception here can be misleading.

A common form of insomnia comes from having high levels of adrenaline, commonly referred to as being an adrenaline junkie. In other words, you have so many stimulating and exciting things going on in your life that your adrenaline never lets up. And with high adrenaline comes reduced need for sleep—a vicious, repeating cycle. No sleep, increased stress. Increased stress, no sleep—over and over again. That's what adrenaline is designed to do: keep us awake to deal with the current demand or emergency.

In fact, you might feel pretty good when you're pumped up on adrenaline. But this feeling sends a false message. You don't feel tired because adrenaline is boosting your alertness and energy. But this system is designed for short-term use only. The price your family will pay for an excessive and prolonged use of their adrenal system is not only sleep deprivation, but a host of health and emotional problems as well.

Parents Need to Be on the Lookout for Sleep Disorders

One of the biggest mistakes a parent can make is to ignore his or her child's sleep problem and assume that it will just go away. Parents need to be on the lookout for the warning signs of a possible sleep disorder and then take action. Very often it masquerades as something else in the early stages. Here are some of the signs to look for in your child:

- Falling asleep in class
- Increase in irritability
- Increase in moodiness or seemingly depressed
- Temper tantrums
- The tendency to emotionally "explode" at the slightest provocation
- Overactivity and hyperactive behavior (restless, fidgety, etc.)
- Falling asleep at home
- Grogginess when waking up in the morning
- Reluctance to wake up or get out of bed in the morning

This is what happened to one family I know. When their son, let's call him Aubrey, was about seven years old, he began to show signs of difficulty in concentrating. If Dad sat down to read a book with him, Aubrey would quickly be distracted by a bird outside or by what his older brother was doing. He also seemed to be tired all the time. Getting him ready for school was a major challenge. First, he wouldn't get out of bed. Then he would yawn a lot, put his head on the kitchen table during breakfast, and fall asleep again. He was teased a lot by other boys at school for being lazy, and he got angry easily. Bottom line, he just didn't want to learn. He ended up being labeled by school officials as having Attention Deficit Disorder (ADD), and for the next four years, doctors tried every medication available for ADD. Finally, his parents began to wonder if there wasn't another cause for his perpetual tiredness. He appeared drowsy almost every day, all day; and no child could possibly learn anything with such a problem.

To some extent, Aubrey's symptoms did fit the profile of ADD. Take note that I'm definitely not saying that parents with ADD children should drop current treatment. But when there is severe tiredness, the problem needs to be investigated further. There are several reasons why a child might manifest symptoms that resemble ADD, but sleep problems should be ruled out before introducing ADD medications. These are usually powerful brain stimulants, which are not without side effects. Over the years, I have encountered many such cases, and it's alarming to consider how inappropriate it was to have these children on powerful drugs when the problem was more basic.

It was Aubrey's vigilant and inquisitive mother who discovered the cause of his problem. Suspecting that Aubrey may have a sleep problem, she took him to a sleep specialist and had his sleep patterns evaluated. The specialist discovered that Aubrey suffered from narcolepsy, a condition that causes undesirable sleepiness at inappropriate times. Inadequate sleep was the real problem that needed to be treated.

(Note: Parents who want to explore the problem of over-medicating children with ADD or ADHD should take a look at a PBS *Frontline* program called "The Medicated Child."[9])

Insomnia and Your Family

As a starting point, remember that insomnia is not a disease. It is a symptom that can have many causes, including bad sleeping habits or a physical disorder. If your spouse or child is having difficulty sleeping, he or she may have a medical or emotional disorder, such as anxiety or depression, or be experiencing too much stress. If this is the case, these problems need to be ruled out first. Make sure your family member has had a complete physical evaluation before proceeding.

If your family member is suffering from a serious sleep deficit, you may need to consult a sleep clinic for evaluation, diagnosis, and treatment. Any of the following symptoms may suggest that you need a sleep laboratory's evaluation:

- Excessive daytime sleepiness or falling asleep uncontrollably
- Continuous insomnia
- Prolonged dependence on sleep aids or pills
- Severe snoring or choking while sleeping
- Repeated and frequent nightmares or night terrors
- If you just feel that there is something abnormal about your family member's sleep pattern

What should you expect to happen at a sleep laboratory?

- A thorough history taken of your sleeping pattern, possibly using a sleep diary like the one I will present later
- A general medical evaluation and history of illnesses
- A few blood tests (to ensure that there are no hormonal problems)
- Possibly a laboratory sleep evaluation where you will be required to sleep over (called an "overnight polysomnography"). Usually you will spend just one night in the lab and sleep with electrodes attached to your head to record brain waves.

The information gathered this way will identify your sleep stages, their duration and interruptions, and your heart rate and breathing patterns. This evaluation will also detect any signs of sleep apnea and possible sleep-movement disorders.

Yes, this is all inconvenient and might even seem like overkill to busy people, but it's the only way to accurately identify a serious sleep disorder. I know many who have been very thankful for what such a thorough evaluation has discovered. Furthermore, it will take the guesswork out of your treatment and speed your recovery time.

Types of Sleepers

Assuming that your or your family member's sleep problem is not serious enough to warrant an overnight polysomnography, the next step is to identify what type of sleeper you or your loved ones are. You've heard the expression, "Oh, I'm a morning person," or "I'm a night person." Morning people like to go to bed early and then get up early. Night people want to stay up late into the night and then sleep in the next day. They prefer to work late and sleep late. Night people usually suffer from not getting enough sleep because they have wasted their most precious sleep time: darkness.

Are there morning people and evening people? Probably. But these traits are not born into us; they are habits we develop. Sorry to burst your bubble here, but hiding behind the belief that you were born to be a "night person" just doesn't work. You are a night person because you have shaped your habits for late-night activities. And like all habits, they can be changed!

How Well Is Your Family Sleeping?

To help you determine whether you or your family members are getting enough sleep, I have put together several assessment tools. You can photocopy them and have each member of your family fill them out. It will help in the evaluation of their sleep habits. For very young children, adapt them as appropriate to their age and fill them in yourself.

1. Evaluate Your Daytime Sleepiness

First, here is an instrument that can help you monitor your daytime doziness and identify its causes. We all experience feeling tired periodically. But which of the following situations make you dozy? Use the following scale by circling the number next to the question that best describes what makes you sleepy:

    0 = no chance of dozing

    1 = slight chance of dozing (once in a while)

    2 = moderate chance of dozing (once a week)

    3 = high chance of dozing (every time)

Circumstance	Chance of becoming dozy
1. Watching television or listening to music	0 1 2 3
2. At the movies or in a theater	0 1 2 3
3. While having a conversation with a family member or friend	0 1 2 3
4. While reading the newspaper or a book	0 1 2 3
5. At work, especially in the afternoon	0 1 2 3
6. Traveling on the bus, on the train, or as a car passenger	0 1 2 3
7. In a waiting room before an appointment	0 1 2 3
8. When driving but stopped in traffic	0 1 2 3
9. Sitting in church, synagogue, or other public places	0 1 2 3
10. Just relaxing	0 1 2 3

Now check your sleepiness score by totaling the points you have given yourself:

Score from 1 to 6: It appears that you are getting enough sleep.

Score from 7 to 10: Your score is above average, but you are starting to show signs of inappropriate drowsiness.

Score of 11 or more: You need to explore further whether you are sleep deprived or have a sleep problem.

2. Evaluate Your Regular Sleep Habits

Now let's do an assessment of your general sleep routine. Here again, adapt the scale to suit a younger age. We will explore how you sleep, for how long, and what the quality of your sleep is like. The assessment tool is designed to bring together key features of your sleep habits so that as we discuss them later, you will know where you are deficient and need to change.

Instructions: For most of your nights, rate the following characteristics of your sleep. There is no scoring here, so merely make a copy of this assessment tool and underline all that apply to you. Remember, underline the appropriate answers so you can review them later. Also, take this evaluation with you if you have to go to a sleep clinic.

Underline the answer that best describes your situation.

1. How many hours do you sleep most nights?

   6 or less; 6 to 7; 7 to 8; 8 to 9; 9 to 10; over 10 hours

2. How often do you consume caffeinated drinks (coffee, colas, etc.)?

   Hardly ever; only in the morning; midday; morning and midday; all through the day

3. How many cups of caffeinated drinks do you consume in a typical day?

4. How do you usually wake up in the morning?

   Naturally; someone wakes me; alarm clock; I have to be shaken

5. How easily do normal night noises wake you?

   Not at all; once a month; once a week; every night

6. What is your sleeping environment like? (Underline *all* that apply.)
   Comfortable; quiet; cozy; restful; conducive to sleep; right heat/cool; dark

7. How often do you exercise moderately?
   Never; once a month; once a week; several times a week; every day

8. Is your level of exercise appropriate for your age and gender?
   Yes; no; maybe; don't know; don't care because it's all I can do

9. What do you do when you can't fall asleep?
   Count sheep (or similar); listen to music; watch TV; read; get up; nothing

10. What do you usually use to help you fall asleep most of the time?
    Don't need help; prayer; meditation; relaxation; take a bath/shower; sleeping pill

11. What time do you usually have to get up on a workday?
    Before 5 AM; 5 to 6 AM; 6 to 7 AM; after 7 AM

12. What do you usually do right before you go to bed? (Underline all you do.)
    Work; exercise; watch TV; read a book; listen to music; play games; bathe or shower; relax in a Jacuzzi; go for a walk/run; sit and talk; surf the Internet

13. Do you ever have to do shift work?
    Yes; no; occasionally

14. Do you go to bed at the same time every night (within a half-hour variation)? Yes; no

15. How often do you nap in the middle of the day?
    Never; once in a while; weekends; 2 or 3 times a week; every day

16. How often have you made an error at work because you were tired?

Never; seldom; once a month; once a week; once a day;
several times a day

17. Have you ever fallen asleep while driving?
Never; occasionally; often for a short period; had an accident
asleep

18. Have you consulted a sleep specialist? Yes; no

19. How often do you take a sleeping pill or other sleep aid?
Every night; once a week; once a month; occasionally; hardly ever
Is it a prescription sleeping pill? Yes; no

20. How many times do you typically wake up during the night?
0; 1 or 2 times; 3 to 5 times; more than 6 times

Closing

While I need to sound a clear warning about the hazards of your family not getting enough sleep, it's not my intention to be an alarmist. I certainly don't want to cause any further disruption to your sleep time by giving you more to worry about. But the statistics supporting the seriousness of our sleep deprivation are indisputable. Almost every day, one reads reports of how sleep deprivation can cause accidental overdoses, car and train accidents, and impaired judgment that can affect many areas of life. Findings like these highlight the danger inherent in our busy, modern lifestyles. It's time for change, and the place to start is in your own life and family.

Determining Your Family's Sleep Habits

It appears that every man's insomnia
is as different from his neighbour's
as are their daytime hopes and aspirations.
—F. SCOTT FITZGERALD

This is essentially a working chapter—a "Discovery Chapter" if you will. Because you need to have a clear understanding of not only your family's sleep problems, but their sleep habits as well. Often, a sleep habit results in a sleep disorder.

Determining Habits That Hinder Sleep

No two families have the same habit patterns, so you need to work through the following exercises yourselves. Just being able to identify and attend to the habits that undermine your ability to get good sleep can help put your family on the road to recovery.

So, following are a series of assessment tools that can help you gather the information you need to identify your and your family's sleep habits and hindrances. Working through these assessment tools will also help you gather important information that can be helpful if you need to consult a sleep specialist.

First, you need to pay particular attention to three factors in assessing the quality of your sleep:

1. Sleep Latency (how quickly you fall asleep): According to the American Academy of Sleep Medicine, for adequate sleep you should be able to fall asleep within 15 minutes of going to bed.[1] If you lose sleep at the start of the night, you will have less sleep the rest of the night, unless you can sleep in and make up what you've lost.

But as important as this point is, let's first be clear about what "falling asleep" means. It does not mean falling immediately into an unconscious state of sleep. The point where you become unconscious is difficult to pinpoint. Also, as I have already pointed out, you may still be aware of what's going on around you during the first two stages of sleep. So don't start your stopwatch and try to time your sleep latency. It will just keep you awake! However, if you sense that you are tossing and turning a lot, and an hour goes by without having fallen asleep, you probably have a sleep latency problem.

2. Sleep Duration: This is the percentage of time you spend in bed actually sleeping. You should be able to stay asleep for 85 percent of the time you are in bed. Here again, don't try to time it. In fact, you may want to turn your clock away from your line of sight so as not to be too distracted by it.

3. Total Sleep Time: As previously mentioned, most experts recommend an optimum of eight or eight and a half hours of sleep a night—minimum! There are some, myself included, who believe that a total sleep time of nine hours is better, for several reasons. First, since we sleep in cycles of about one and a half hours and our dream sleep comes at or near the end of each cycle, it just makes sense that the total sleep time for a normal and healthy adult should be a multiple of one and a half hours. For children, of course, it should be longer. We need to complete each sleep cycle of 90 minutes in order to reap the full benefits. Cutting the last cycle short doesn't make sense. This means

that our total sleep time options, using multiples of one and a half hours, are as follows:

Option 1: Four and a half hours. (A bad idea—it will kill you eventually.)

Option 2: Six hours. (Better, but still dangerous.)

Option 3: Seven and a half hours. (Where most are now, but not enough for a healthy brain.)

Option 4: Nine hours. (Now we're making sense.)

Option 5: Ten and a half hours. (Typical for Type B people and those who are sick and need more rest. Longer than this may indicate a health problem. Although, I have found that many normal people need more sleep even than this.)

A second reason why total sleep time should be nine hours revolves around how we define "sleep duration." If you ask the average person how long he or she sleeps, he's bound to report how long it is he thinks he was unconscious. And since we have no idea when we become unconscious, the answer is invariably inaccurate. Also, since we sleep in stages, some stages are so light that you may feel you are still awake. This is why I prefer to define sleep duration as the total amount of time spent in bed. This removes any confusion. Part of this time is just resting our bodies. Part of the time we are in a light sleep, and then for the remainder we are in a deep sleep. Finally, we dream and then return to one of the previous stages—often waking up. So don't get sidetracked into thinking that you are only sleeping when you are unconscious.

In setting a target for your total sleep time, therefore, you should aim for a sleep duration that you know helps you function at your best. This, and only this criterion, should guide you. Forget about whether you think others get less or more sleep than yourself. Just find out what suits you best.

The following questionnaire will help to capture and summarize your baseline sleep habits. There are no right or wrong answers. It merely puts all the information together in such a way that you can get a good overview of your sleep pattern. This record will be helpful for your doctor should you seek professional help. As with all the tools I offer, I recommend making photocopies of the pages. By making several copies, you can retake the questionnaires at several-week intervals and monitor your progress, or pass them on to someone else and give him or her the chance to use the assessment tools.

As you continue to read this book, keep this sleep assessment close by so you can evaluate your own sleeping pattern, or that of a family member. Taking this assessment again later, after you have made some sleep changes, will help you see how much progress you have made.

Baseline Sleep Questionnaire
(Underline all the answers, or fill in the blanks,
that describe your daily sleep habits.)

1. About how many hours sleep do you get most nights?
   9 or more; 8; 7; 6; less than 6
2. How many cups of regular coffee or other caffeinated drinks do you drink a day? _____
3. When do you drink caffeinated drinks?
   Morning; midday; evening; all day
4. How do you wake up in the morning?
   Naturally; alarm clock; someone wakes me
5. How easily do night noises wake you?
   Not at all; once or twice a night; often
6. Is your sleep environment conducive to good sleep? Yes / No
7. How often do you exercise?
   Never; once a week; several times a week; every day
8. What sort of thoughts keep you awake?
   Personal; family; work; illness; other: _____

9. What helps you fall asleep?
    Don't need help; prayer/meditate; relax; a bath;
    other: _____

10. What time do you usually go to bed on a weeknight?
    _____ AM/PM

11. What time do you usually go to bed on the weekend?
    _____ AM/PM

12. What time do you usually have to get up on a workday?
    _____ AM/PM

13. What time do you usually have to get up on the weekend?
    _____ AM/PM

14. Do you ever have to do shift work? Yes / No

15. How often do you nap in the middle of the day?
    Never; once or more a week; every day

16. How often have you made an error at work because you were
    tired?
    Never; a few times; many times

17. Do you go to bed pretty much at the same time every night?
    Yes / No

18. How dark is your bedroom?
    Dark; somewhat dark; not dark at all

19. How silent is your neighborhood at night?
    Quiet; somewhat noisy; noisy

20. Are you totally satisfied with your sleep time and habits?
    Yes / No

In addition to this Baseline Sleep Questionnaire, you should also keep a summary of your mood and energy level. Your mood and energy levels are helpful indicators of the effects sleep deprivation might be having on your daily life. The following is not a test, but merely a way of recording how your (or your family's) mood and energy fluctuate from day to day.

Basic Mood and Energy Questionnaire

Instructions: This questionnaire should be filled in at the end of each day, over a period of at least one week. Record your mood and energy by placing a check mark after the number shown that best describes how you have felt for most of the day or the period stated.

> 0 – I did not have this feeling
>
> 1 – I felt it slightly
>
> 2 – I felt it moderately
>
> 3 – I felt it very strongly
>
> 4 – I felt it strongly

Date (Start of week): ___ / ___ / ___ Day of week: (Circle) Monday, Tuesday, Wednesday, Thursday, Friday, Saturday, Sunday

1. I felt energetic when I woke up this morning.

    0 __ 1 __ 2 __ 3 __ 4 __

2. At midday I felt energetic.

    0 __ 1 __ 2 __ 3 __ 4 __

3. At the end of the workday I felt energetic.

    0 __ 1 __ 2 __ 3 __ 4 __

4. I felt energetic at bedtime.

    0 __ 1 __ 2 __ 3 __ 4 __

5. My mood was upbeat when I woke up.

    0 __ 1 __ 2 __ 3 __ 4 __

6. My mood was upbeat at midday.

    0 __ 1 __ 2 __ 3 __ 4 __

7. My mood was upbeat at the end of the workday.

    0 __ 1 __ 2 __ 3 __ 4 __

8. My mood was upbeat when I went to bed.

    0 __ 1 __ 2 __ 3 __ 4 __

9. I felt irritable when I woke up.

    0 __ 1 __ 2 __ 3 __ 4 __

10. I felt irritable at midday.
   0 __ 1 __ 2 __ 3 __ 4 __

11. I felt irritable at the end of the workday.
   0 __ 1 __ 2 __ 3 __ 4 __

12. I felt irritable when I went to bed.
   0 __ 1 __ 2 __ 3 __ 4 __

File each day's record away so you can use it in conjunction with the sleep diary I will describe next.

Keeping a Sleep Diary

You can learn a lot about your sleep patterns and habits by keeping a daily sleep diary. If other members of your family are having difficulty sleeping, encourage them to begin a sleep diary as well. There are many forms of sleep diaries available on the Internet, but you can easily create one for yourself. You simply need a chart that will keep a record of the following:

- The time you went to bed and woke up
- How long and well you slept
- When you were awake during the night
- How much caffeine or alcohol you consumed and when
- What/when you ate and drank
- What emotion or stress you had
- What drugs or medications you took

I have prepared two such diaries for your use, which can be found in Appendix A and Appendix B. The first (Appendix A: Sleep Diary Part One) is to be filled out in the morning, right after you wake up, and the second in the evening, just before you go to bed. Make several copies of each. Make a record of your sleep pattern before you start to change anything, and then repeat the diary at a later time so you can compare the two records and see where you have improved. These records can also help you see whether or not your change strategies are working.

Notice that the diary asks you to fill in information about when you went to bed, approximately fell asleep, got up, and woke up during the night, if you did so at all. This is important because it will identify whether or not your sleeping is being interrupted each night at the same time. And if it is, you can begin to explore what it is that is waking you up.

I had a patient who did this and discovered she was waking up at the same time every night. So she decided to make a continuous tape recording of the night. It was back in the days when you could get long recording tapes and machines with slow recording speeds. To her surprise she found that it was her husband's snoring that would wake her up. No, she didn't kick him out of the bedroom. It only took a couple of earplugs to rectify the matter. But it could have just as easily been a neighbor's dog or a noisy refrigerator. Whatever is disrupting your sleep needs to be identified and dealt with.

The second diary (Appendix B: Sleep Diary Part Two) is to be filled out just before going to bed. Here you will record the activities of your day that might be affecting your sleep. You should record how much caffeine you took in (coffee and other drinks), what medications you are taking (some of them can affect your sleep), whether and when you exercised (it might help to change the amount and time of your exercising), and what other activities you engaged in during the day that might have affected your sleep.

And since the topic of having sex late at night might be on some readers' minds (I get asked about it often), let me hasten to add that sex is not usually a sleep inhibitor. In fact, it's quite the opposite. It can release tension and act as a tranquilizer. Extreme forms of sex (activity normally considered to be perverse, such as extreme cruelty or asphyxia while sexually aroused) are another matter and can act as an adrenaline stimulant.

You can also use these sleep diaries to record your teens' and children's sleeping habits. Teens can fill it in for themselves, but you may have to do it for your children by asking them key questions.

After you have collected at least a week's data for your sleep diary, you are ready to do some analyzing. If you have spreadsheet computer skills, you might want to transfer the data to a spreadsheet so you can get a better overview of your sleep habits. On your spreadsheet or summary sheet, you can also combine data from other inventories in the book, especially those that record how you feel each day. This will immediately help you to see how your mood and general state of mind are being affected after, say a bad night, or alternatively, how much better you feel after a good night's sleep.

As you review your sleep diary, you will notice that some nights you sleep more or better than others, and that your energy and mood levels will fluctuate up or down. What cause and effect can you identify? To help find the answer, ask yourself the following questions and jot down some notes about it so you can review your thoughts later:

1. Why am I getting more and better sleep some nights and not on others? Are there any habits that always precede a bad night's sleep? (For instance, pay attention to your caffeine intake—both when you take it and how much you take in. Does it show up in altered sleep patterns?)

2. What effect does my sleep have on my energy level and general mood the next day? Are there any clear patterns here? Is there a clear connection between how much I sleep and my energy level? (Also, try varying the amount of time you sleep—for example, go to bed earlier and then note the changes it makes to your mood and energy level the next day.)

3. Am I consistently getting enough sleep each night or does it vary? If not, what does my diary tell me about what is preventing it?

4. What sort of activities are affecting how much I sleep and the quality of my sleep? (If you keep the diary going long enough, you might

be surprised by how much you are missing or not attending to in your life that could have an effect on your sleep. It's easy to deny or ignore something obvious that could easily be rectified, if only you were aware of it.)

5. What sort of habits can I change to ensure I am getting enough sleep to function well and feel better? Avoiding caffeine? Asking my doctor to try some form of medication? Going to bed earlier? Getting up later? Changing my mattress or pillow? Using earplugs? Changing eating habits, such as eating my main meal at lunchtime? Improving my airconditioning? Adding more time to my in-bed time?

After you've made any changes, take a diary record again to see how much you have improved.

The following Sleepiness Scale will help you identify situations that tend to reveal your level of sleepiness. Strictly speaking, none of these situations should make you go to sleep if you are adequately rested.

Sleepiness Scale

Instructions: Use the following scale and place a number that best fits your response next to each question.

0 = Never doze

1 = Sometimes doze

2 = Often doze

1. Sitting and reading: _____

2. Watching TV: _____

3. Sitting inactive in a public place (e.g., church):   _____

4. As a passenger in a car: _____

5. Lying down to rest in the afternoon: _____

6. Sitting and talking to someone: _____

7. Sitting quietly after a lunch: _____

8. In a social setting (friends visiting):   _____

9. In a theatre during a movie: ____
10. During lectures or speeches: ____

TOTAL ____

SCORING: Total the ratings. The maximum score possible is 20.

Interpretation:

- If your score is less than 5, you are most likely getting an adequate amount of sleep.
- If your score is between 5 and 8, you need to take steps to improve your sleeping.
- If your score is between 9 and 12, you need to consult a sleep specialist right away.
- If your score is greater than 13, you need to talk to your health care provider right away because you may have a sleep disorder. Make a copy of this questionnaire and your answers and discuss them with the doctor.

So, since this is a discovery chapter, how can you tell if you need more sleep? In addition to avoiding the sleep killers I have already discussed, here is some information that might help you evaluate whether your sleep is sufficient. (The statistics quoted come from a poll conducted by the National Sleep Foundation titled "Women and Sleep Today"[2] but is equally applicable to both men and women.)

1. Do you feel refreshed when you wake up in the morning? Fifty-eight percent of stay-at-home moms, 56 percent of moms who work full-time, and 41 percent of moms who work part-time do not wake up feeling refreshed at least a few days every week. Not waking up feeling refreshed is mostly a sign of lack of sleep.

2. Do you ever have trouble falling asleep or staying asleep? Seventy-four percent of stay-at-home moms, 72 percent of full-time working moms, and 60 percent of part-time working moms experience symptoms of insomnia a few nights a week.

3. Does snoring keep you or your loved ones awake? One-third of women snore at least a few nights a week. We might joke and make light of it, but it is a classic symptom of sleep apnea, a serious and potentially life-threatening sleep disorder if left untreated. Many women are also kept awake by their partner's snoring and suffer as a result. Later in the book, I offer some practical suggestions and steps to prevent it from bothering you.

4. Do you have nighttime disturbances such as children, pets, needing to go to the bathroom, pain, stress, nightmares, and so on? You need to be assertive in finding solutions. Don't settle into a learned helplessness mode of existence.

5. Are you experiencing a decline in your sex life? Lack of sleep will affect virtually every aspect of your life, including your sex life. Forty-four percent of full-time working moms, 39 percent of stay-at-home moms, and 28 percent of part-time working moms say they are too tired for sex. In a study my oldest daughter and I conducted of women across the U.S., women reported losing their libido for at least a few years after giving birth to their second child.[3] Husbands need to understand this, and couples need to find a way around it. It's just an idea, but getting more sleep might just work some miracles here!

Menopause and Sleep Problems

I have a special reason for including a brief discussion about menopause as a sleep disrupter. No, I am not menopausal! My wife runs a pastors' wives support group in our area, and over the past few months she has heard from many wives who tell her how their menopause has robbed them of sleep. When one of the ladies heard I was writing a book about sleep, she immediately e-mailed me the following: "If the book has a section dealing with menopause and sleep, I'll buy it!" So how could I possibly overlook this topic? The sale of one book is at stake!

One of the most illuminating findings in recent sleep research is how menopause can affect a woman's sleep. Menopause typically occurs in the late forties to early fifties, although there is evidence that it is now starting earlier, just as the age of puberty is starting earlier.

If you have menopausal-related sleep problems, you need to check with your physician on how to best manage this time in your life. Treating the symptoms of menopause can help. Previously, the traditional treatment was hormone replacement therapy (HRT). HRT consisted of estrogen given as a pill, patch, or vaginal cream, either used alone or combined with progesterone (for women who still have their utcrus). But then it was discovered that the long-term use of estrogen-progesterone combination therapy caused an increased risk of breast cancer, heart disease, blood clots, and stroke. Estrogen alone did not increase breast cancer or heart disease, but the study found that therapy with estrogen alone did increase the risk of blood clots and stroke and uterine cancer.

So the latest recommendation for use of HRT for severe menopause symptoms is to use the lowest possible dose for the shortest possible period, and then have a regular follow-up with your doctor.

As far as sleeping better is concerned, hot flashes are a common interruption. The following suggestions might help you keep cooler at night and sleep better without the use of hormonal supplements:

1. Wear loose clothing to bed. When you sweat you need lots of room so your skin can breathe.

2. Keep your bedroom cool and well ventilated. Your spouse may need to go and sleep in the spare room for a while.

3. Avoid foods that may cause sweating (such as spicy foods), especially right before bedtime.

4. Maintain a regular bedtime schedule. Managing your diurnal clock is difficult enough without further aggravations!

5. Exercise regularly, but not right before going to bed, as this will make you sweat. If possible, midday is the best time to exercise.

6. Avoid excessive caffeine, including chocolates. Sorry about this, but it will only aggravate the problem!

7. Avoid deep sleep during the day, as this can prevent you from sleeping well at night. Of course, if you are sleep deprived, then an afternoon sleep (not just a nap) can make up the shortfall, but for the most part, save that deep sleep for nighttime.

Avoiding Hazardous Sleep Disorders

When thou liest down, thou shalt not be afraid:
yea, thou shalt lie down, and thy sleep shall be sweet.
—PROVERBS 3:24 (KJV)

As we have already seen, sleep deprivation is not just an innocent intruder. Almost every week, reports come across my desk that illustrate the serious consequences of sleep deprivation. One report I read was about a 13-year-old girl who kept falling asleep in school. Because she didn't want to be ridiculed, she tried to hide her sleepiness from her friends. She was even too embarrassed to tell her own mother, for fear she would be labeled as lazy.

Finally, after she had fallen asleep standing at a bus stop and nearly fell over in front of an approaching bus, she did tell her mother that she felt something was wrong. Her mother admitted noticing that her daughter would fall asleep at odd times, like at the dinner table or just watching TV, but she had just put it down to teenage fatigue and languor, and ignored it.

But at this point, she took her daughter to a sleep specialist. An overnight sleep study revealed that the young girl suffered from sleep apnea, a disorder where someone wakes up at night because he or she stops breathing due to partial obstruction of the airway. The sleep interruptions that come with sleep apnea can create a severe and dangerous state of sleep deprivation that can affect daytime functioning.

One of the reasons why disorders such as sleep apnea often go unnoticed in young people is that children and teens don't always show the usual signs that adults do, like deep snoring or choking. Most children with the disorder, and their parents, aren't even aware of the frequent awakenings during the night. The child is usually too tired to wake up entirely and in the morning does not recall waking up throughout the night.

And for many, sleep deprivation, though troubling, is not necessarily life threatening. But this is not true for all. A recent CBS News report said that 12 million Americans suffer from nightly attacks of interrupted, oxygen-deprived sleep (sleep apnea). According to a new study by Johns Hopkins University, sleep apnea raises the risk of death from all causes, for middle-aged and elderly people, by as much as 46 percent in the most severe cases, and 17 percent in moderate cases.[1] The study is a landmark in sleep-apnea research because it quantifies the risk of death that the medical community has always known existed.

But many dangerous sleep disorders, like sleep apnea, go unrecognized or untreated. So I would be remiss if I did not discuss, albeit briefly, those forms of sleep disruption or deprivation that can threaten life itself. These disorders require professional help, and while I will offer some suggestions for alleviating them, you should seek professional treatment right away if you think you have any of the serious disorders I mention.

Without a doubt, some mild sleep disorders can also be dangerous. It's dangerous to drive a vehicle or work heavy machinery when you haven't had a good night's sleep. But I want to go beyond this and sound a warning about other, more serious emotional hazards of sleep deprivation. Serious mental disorders, including clinical depression and rage, can readily be triggered during times of sleeplessness.[2] So can suicide.

While sleep deprivation itself may not be the cause of a suicide, if someone is suicidal, sleeplessness increases the sufferer's confusion and could be the trigger of a suicidal, or homicidal, act.

Quite by coincidence, shortly after starting to write this book, I received several letters from parents of young men and women who had recently committed suicide. Common to all these letters was one theme: The suicide of their beloved family members had followed an obvious period of sleep deprivation.

Pay Careful Attention to Sleeplessness

I have pointed out that there's a tendency these days to trivialize the seriousness of sleep deprivation and shrug it off with a casual, "Well, everyone struggles to get enough sleep, so my problem is no big deal." Perhaps *your* problem is not serious, but for others in your family, trouble sleeping can have a severe penalty. So parents of teenagers and young adults should pay careful attention here. This age group is at high risk for depression and vulnerable to sleep loss because their bodies and minds need more sleep, not less. In fact, children as young as three years old are being diagnosed with clinical depression, according to a recent Associated Press news report.[3] This is alarming, because until recently we didn't believe children that young could suffer from clinical depression. What is the suspected cause? Yes, you guessed it—insufficient sleep.

A national survey published by the *New England Journal of Medicine* in 2005, found that of 13,500 college students surveyed, almost 45 percent reported being so depressed that they had difficulty functioning, and 94 percent reported feeling confused and overwhelmed by everything they had to do.[4] While many of these students may not actually meet the criteria for clinical depression, their self-perceived mood clearly speaks for itself. It's critical that parents pay close attention to their teens' and children's sleeping habits as well, as these will impact both the cause of depression as well as how well they cope with it. A child who develops bad sleeping habits is likely to carry these habits over into adolescence and adulthood.

A Brief Review of the More Serious Sleep Disorders

Lured by thousands of scientific presentations, 10,000 neurologists and neuroscientists attended the 59th annual meeting of the American Academy of Neurology in May 2007. Their focus was on sleep disorders in our time. Over one hundred presentations documented research on a variety of sleep disorders, including the effects of socioeconomic status on children's sleeping habits (poor neighborhoods often can't provide good sleep hygiene because of overcrowding), the influence of sleep apnea on the human immune response, the decline of cognitive function in elderly women, and several interesting papers on restless legs syndrome (RLS).

All told, it was an impressive conference and highlighted the seriousness and breadth of our sleep problems. Much of what follows comes from the findings presented at this conference. I will examine each of the more serious sleep disorders confronting us today, help you determine whether you have any of these problems, and then point the way to some solutions.

Dangerous Sleep Disorders

The Greek word *apnea* literally means "without breath."[5] So sleep apnea is a disorder in which you are not breathing while sleeping. When this happens, a sensor in the brain shocks the system into wakefulness as soon as it detects lowered oxygen.

There are three types of sleep apnea:

1. Obstructive (the airway is being blocked)
2. Central (the brain isn't sending a signal telling your body to breathe)
3. Mixed (some of both)

Obstructive sleep apnea (OSA), sometimes aptly called the "Phantom of the Night," is the most common form of sleep apnea and is caused when the soft tissue at the rear of the throat collapses and closes the airway during sleep. In central sleep apnea the airway is not blocked, but the brain fails to signal the muscles to breathe. This is a much more serious condition that requires seeing a neurologist immediately.

The sudden waking by the brain with each apnea event can be quite a shock to the system. And it can happen as many as 15 times an hour. Needless to say, this leaves the sufferer exhausted, unslept, and brain-befuddled. The sufferer is not always aware that he or she has temporarily stopped breathing, or may discount it. Often, it's the spouse who draws attention to it.

Sleep apnea is almost as common as diabetes. It affects more than 12 million Americans, according to the National Institutes of Health. Risk factors include being a male (I've always suspected that there's a downside to being a man), being overweight (get back to doing your exercises and eat well), and being over 40 (this is when muscles in the throat start to sag). Obese elderly men are at greatest risk, but sleep apnea can strike anyone at any age.

Untreated, sleep apnea will likely cause severe sleep disruption. It can also cause high blood pressure, memory problems, weight gain, impotence, strokes, heart attacks, and headaches. It may be responsible for job impairment and motor vehicle crashes. Fortunately, sleep apnea can be diagnosed and treated. Several treatment options exist, and research into additional options continues even as I'm writing.

Since it's the tissue at the back of the throat that drops during sleep and shuts off the airway, recent studies have indicated that loud snoring doesn't just annoy a spouse; it can signal sleep apnea. The culprit is the flabby tissue at the back of the throat that causes the snoring. It is now so common that Medicare is considering allowing at-home testing for sleep apnea, letting people snooze in their own beds instead of spending the night in a strange sleep clinic or laboratory.[6]

If, perchance, you do have sleep apnea, here are your major treatment options:

- Continuous Positive Airway Pressure (CPAP for short): This is a common treatment for more serious apneas. A small portable machine gently blows pressurized room air through your airway at a pressure high enough to keep the back of your throat open. The pressure is set according to your oxygen level and eliminates the apneas that cause frequent awakenings. Since you have to sleep with a mask on your face, it may take a few nights or even weeks to get used to it.

- Oral Appliances: Dental appliances can treat apnea by keeping the airway open in several ways: by pushing the lower jaw forward, by preventing the tongue from falling back over the airway (a tongue-retaining device), or by combining both. Oral appliances are typically more effective for people with mild sleep apnea and for non-obese people, but can also be effective for moderate and severe sleep apnea. Ask your doctor to refer you to a dentist who is familiar with sleep apnea and who works with oral appliances. A friend of mine has recently developed a very effective dental device that can help relieve sleep apnea and snoring. It is called the FAEBS. Its uniqueness is that the upper and lower parts of the device can move in any direction, so it has a more natural feel in the mouth and is more tolerable.

Sleep Apnea Assessment Scale

While a yes to a simple question like "Do you snore and gasp at night while sleeping on a regular basis?" is enough for you to suspect sleep apnea, the following questionnaire might identify more subtle forms of this disorder.

Circle either Yes or No in response to the following questions:

1. Do you wake up with headaches most mornings? Yes/No
2. Do you often wake up feeling tired, foggy, or not ready to face the day? Yes/No
3. Do you fall asleep easily during the day? Yes/No
4. Are you overweight? Yes/No
5. Do you have high blood pressure? Yes/No
6. Do you have trouble breathing through your nose? Yes/No
7. Do you snore loudly when sleeping? Yes/No
8. Do you have to sleep propped up with pillows or sitting up? Yes/No
9. Have you fallen out of bed more than once or twice? Yes/No
10. Are you restless when you sleep, tossing to and fro or turning frequently? Yes/No

Only a professional can diagnose sleep apnea with certainty. But if you have answered Yes to two or more of questions 1 to 5, and Yes to one or more of questions 6 to 10, you need to consult your doctor and request a test for sleep apnea right away.

- Positional Therapy: This is effective only in less serious cases. Since sleeping on the back worsens apnea, not sleeping on the back may reduce the number of apneas. To avoid sleeping on their backs, some people use homemade gadgets like tennis balls in a tube sock attached to the back of the pajamas. A number of companies produce pillows that reduce snoring and mild sleep apnea by positioning the neck so as to open the airway.
- Weight Loss: Additional fat around the neck may make the airway narrower, and obstructions are more likely to occur. So losing weight can reduce the frequency of sleep apnea.
- Avoiding Alcohol: Alcohol and certain medications that act as central nervous system (CNS) depressants, such as painkillers, sedatives, and muscle relaxants, can all worsen sleep apnea by relaxing the airway muscles further. Hence, avoid all alcohol and CNS depressants close to bedtime.
- Surgery: If all else fails, you may need surgery to create a more open airway so obstructions are less likely to occur. There are several surgical procedures, so make sure you talk through all the options and risks with your doctor.

Restless Legs Syndrome (RLS)

This is also called "nocturnal myoclonus" (night-time jerking). It's characterized by uncomfortable sensations that occur mainly in the legs and an irresistible and uncontrollable urge to move one's legs or sometimes one's arms or torso as well. Moving the affected body part provides temporary relief, but the cycle starts all over again.

It's a somewhat contentious disorder. Many physicians claim that the incidence of restless legs syndrome is exaggerated by manufacturers of the drugs used to treat it, but most agree that it is a real problem that has specific diagnostic criteria. I admit to periodically suffering from it myself.

RLS Signs and Symptoms

The restless sensations and pressing need to move one's limbs usually come when lying down. This is why they disturb your sleep. During sleep the legs move spontaneously and uncontrollably, often waking the sleeper. It may start at any age, including early childhood, and become progressive. Between 1 and 5 percent of adults suffer from it.[7] Often the movements increase during times of stress. The sensations are unusual and unlike other common sensations, and those with RLS have a hard time describing them. People use words such as: uncomfortable, antsy, electrical, creeping, painful, itching, pins and needles, pulling, creepy-crawly, ants inside the legs, and many others.

Treatment of RLS

RLS can be aggravated by other medical conditions, such as kidney disease, so it's important that you have a complete medical evaluation to rule out specific causes. Although medications are a common treatment for RLS, no single drug works for everyone. The medications prescribed for restless legs syndrome are frequently "off-label," meaning that they are not specifically approved for RLS, but have been found to help reduce symptoms. The dosage given for RLS is usually much less than the dosage used in other conditions.

Here are some approved medications used to treat RLS:
- Dopaminergic agents—often the same as those used to treat Parkinson's disease.
- Benzodiazepines—tranquilizers used as regular sleep medications. They also suppress muscle contractions.
- Non-benzodiazepine sedatives—short-acting sleeping pills. These may be helpful for mild RLS and aid sleep.
- Opiates—pain-killing medications and relaxing drugs that can suppress RLS in some people. They are addictive and should be used only in low dosages.

• Anticonvulsants (examples: Gabapentin, Neurontin)—normally used to prevent seizures, but can reduce muscle contractions in some people.

Talk with your doctor and be cautious with your use of these drugs. Drug ads may make sleep medications seem effective and safe, but in reality they often work only slightly better than a placebo, while causing major side effects. Additionally, some of these medications may paradoxically increase RLS symptoms, a condition called "augmentation."

Alternative non-drug treatments: Non-drug treatments include exercising the limbs or regular walking, as these can bring immediate relief. Doing stretch exercises, swimming, biking, or other physical activity may also relieve the symptoms. Fast up-and-down movement of the legs, called "sewing machine legs," can keep the restless sensations at bay without your having to actually walk. Try different types of exercise and movements to see which helps you the most.

If you use the relaxation exercises offered in Appendix D, avoid those that involve muscle relaxation, because the relaxation of muscles can sometimes increase the restlessness. Slow breathing or hand-warming exercises might work better.

Hypersomnia

Hypersomnia, as the name suggests, is over-sleeping or excessive tiredness. I suspect that there are some who wouldn't mind occasionally suffering from this disorder. When it follows an illness like the flu, extreme sleepiness brings healing, forcing your body to take time to rest. When it occurs over the weekend or when you are on holiday, it is also quite normal. The adrenaline drop and wind-down helps you catch up on much-needed sleep. But when your sleeping is longer than 25 percent of what you normally sleep, it classifies as "hypersomnia." So if you normally sleep for 8 hours and now find yourself wanting to sleep for 10 hours, and you are not suffering from some illness, it may be a sign that you are experiencing hypersomnia. Since hypersomnia could indicate a more serious disorder, you should seek medical attention.

In narcolepsy (suddenly falling asleep) there are uncontrollable episodes of sleep during normal waking hours, as well as sudden periods of muscle weakness. Narcolepsy is not common, but it tends to run in families, so it is often identified at an early age because other family members are aware of it.

Sleepwalking (Somnambulism)

I rarely get questions about sleepwalking in my seminars. Most sufferers of sleepwalking are too embarrassed to talk about it. But the news media love it. Some reports are quite humorous—to the reader, not the sufferer. A recent news report told the story of one man who woke up early one morning to find himself under his bed, looking for his passport so he could go on vacation. The next morning he woke up to find himself under his bed, looking for his suitcase to go on the imaginary vacation. Then the following night, he successfully found his suitcase and his passport, and woke up while he was packing his clothes! He really worried that he might wake up one day to find himself on an airplane.

But not all sleepwalking escapades are humorous. Some can be quite dangerous. In May 2009, the press reported that a sleepwalking teenager jumped from her bedroom window, 25 feet above the ground.[8] She landed feet first on a strip of grass, leaving six-inch holes in the ground before collapsing. Semi-conscious, she screamed for help. Her parents rushed her to the hospital, and amaxingly, tests revealed she hadn't broken any bones. But that's not the end of the story. It wasn't until the following day that the teenager fully woke up.

From the literature on the topic, it appears that sleepwalking is more common in children than adults, with about 18 percent of children in the United States being prone to sleepwalking, according to the National Academy for Childhood Sleep Disorders.[9] Sleepwalking is more common in boys than girls, and during the ages of 6 to 12 years. Sometimes there is a genetic connection.

"In addition, medical reports from the National Academy for Childhood Sleep Disorders state that if a child continues to sleepwalk after the age of 9, the incidence of sleepwalking in adulthood increases by 75 percent, compared to those children whose sleepwalking activity ceases before the age of nine."[10]

Why is sleepwalking a problem? Well, here again, all sorts of activities can take place during sleepwalking—some quite embarrassing and some, as we have seen, even dangerous. Eating, bathing, urinating, dressing, driving a car, whistling, sexual intercourse, and murder have all been reported during a sleepwalking adventure. No doubt some of these reports are exaggerated, but clearly, if you walk in your sleep, you could injure yourself.

So, what are the facts here? Contrary to popular belief, in most cases of sleepwalking the person does not actually walk around without some conscious knowledge of the behavior. Most sleepwalking occurs after a person is partly awakened (something or someone has disturbed his or her sleep), and the person may just sit up or stand up in a daze, look around for a moment, and then lie back down and fall asleep. Hardly any walking has actually taken place. But these incidents are rarely reported and only go on record if seen during an observation in a sleep clinic. Since it cannot occur during the deepest stage of sleep (you are literally paralyzed), sleepwalking must occur in a light stage of sleep.

Contrary to what is depicted in old-fashioned movies and cartoons, sleepwalkers do not walk around with their eyes closed and arms stretched out. Rather, they engage in activities with their eyes open. (Otherwise how could they navigate their surroundings?) The victim's eyes may have a glazed or empty, far-off appearance, and the subject may be slow or unable to answer or respond in an intelligible manner.

Dealing with Sleepwalking

If you encounter a family member sleepwalking, gently direct the person back to their bed. If it's a small child, you might want to carry him or her back to bed. However, the sleepwalker may get up again if he or she did not yet accomplish the task that prompted the sleepwalking in the first place. For instance, if a sleepwalker is cleaning or sweeping the floor (a common sleepwalking activity), try to assist in the cleaning and so give the person reason to go back to bed. Sleepwalkers tend not to remember anything said or done afterward, so there is no need to worry about embarrassing them at that moment.

Also, remember that sleepwalkers are highly suggestible, so anything they hear or see may trigger a change in behavior. Since sleepwalkers are unaware of what they are doing, they may exhibit awkward behaviors, such as undressing or urinating, which could be embarrassing afterward.

As a general rule, one should not wake a sleepwalker. However, if something dangerous is about to happen, take whatever precautions necessary to prevent harm to anyone, including the sleepwalker. You might want to install a home security system so as to alert you if your child tries to leave the house. Also, make sure that all pools of water, including fish ponds and swimming pools, have protective enclosures with locks, that medications are out of reach, and that fires are extinguished. In other words, remove anything that can harm a child who is prone to sleepwalking. There are no proven treatments for sleepwalking, but it could be helpful to go to a sleep clinic for a complete evaluation to rule out any other sleep disorder.

Nightmares and Night Terrors

This is a common topic, often raised in my seminars. Some call night-mares "dysfunctional dreaming," meaning that they are dreams gone wrong. Frightening dreams usually wake you up, so they are remembered vividly. However, sometimes they don't wake you right away and you recall them only later. They occur during REM sleep and can bring out "feelings of strong fear, terror, distress, or extreme anxiety."[11]

A recent study at the University of the West of England (John Smith, verbal communications, 2009) found that women reported having more nightmares than men—19 percent for men compared to 30 percent for women.[12] The study indicated that menstruation could increase vivid and disturbing dreams. These researchers believed that nightmares help the brain to "rehearse" distressing and disturbing events that one is likely to encounter in the future, so they are, in a sense, necessary.

Three distinct types of nightmares were identified: being chased or haunted; the loss of a parent, child, or partner; and weird and new environments. So the next time you have a nightmare with one of these themes, chalk it up to your brain just doing what it's designed to do!

On the other hand, children seem to have more nightmares than adults. They do have a lot more to be scared about, and the experience can be more distressing. Bad dreams can also be caused by medications, illness, spicy foods, traumatic events (like a car accident), or past traumatic events being remembered. While they can commonly come at any time, not getting enough sleep so that one is so exhausted and stays longer in stage 4 sleep is a common trigger in both adults and children. Usually there is also some underlying stress, a fever, or excessive tiredness acting together to trigger it. In adults, abrupt alcohol withdrawal, sleep apnea, grief, illness with fever, and reaction to the side effects of drugs can trigger nightmares as well.[13]

In a night terror, a person may sit up, scream, and throw him- or herself around in extreme fright. But night terrors are not just bad dreams or nightmares. In fact, a person suffering from a night terror is not even necessarily dreaming, as night terrors can come at any stage of sleep (though they can be triggered by nightmares). Panic attacks can also trigger night terrors, and this is the first cause that needs to be checked out. A sudden onset of regular night terrors, usually coming on at the same time every night, is a sure indicator of panic attacks that are being triggered during sleep.

For some, during a night terror their eyes are wide open, even though they may still be partly asleep. Their hearts are racing, and they may be hyperventilating. They feel overwhelmed by a drive to escape—all similar to panic attacks. But night terrors may not involve any panic symptoms as such. It's more a feeling of terror.

Again, night terrors are more common in children, but they usually stop as the child gets older, say after puberty. If a child does have a night terror and still appears to be sleeping, do not try to wake him. Make sure he is safe and gently return him to the sleeping position. He may not recall the terror afterward, so don't fear any long-term effects. When adults have night terrors, it's usually during a period of intense stress or when having psychological problems. Here, again, alcohol will only aggravate the problem.

Treatment for both night terrors and nightmares usually involves dealing with the underlying problem. The victim may have a fever or be stressed. Several of the long-acting tranquilizers, like clonazepam, as well as some antidepressants, like imipramine, can be helpful in reducing both night terrors and nightmares.

Sleep and the Elderly

Sleep deprivation in the elderly can be particularly hazardous. It can increase dizziness and the risk of falling and disorient someone driving. Helping the elderly manage sleep problems is not as easy as it might seem. There are several reasons for this. Older people experience sleep problems more frequently. For instance, as we age we might sleep less at night, have more nighttime awakenings, and need a second sleep during the day. Also, the deeper stages of sleep may get shorter. The elderly also differ widely in their sleep habits and history. They experience a great variety and increased frequency of health-related problems, all of which can disrupt sleep. Arthritis, for example, can be a real sleep killer. Elderly people are also likely to be taking a variety of medications, and some of these may cause side effects that can disrupt sleep.

How much sleep does an elderly person need? Well, this is also not easily answered. I have heard some experts say that the elderly need less sleep, but that has not been my experience. Some sleep less; others sleep more. Obviously it depends on many factors, so let me explain a few of them because confusion here can increase sleep hazards to the elderly.

Let's suppose that Joe, a former computer programmer who is now retired, has worked mainly with his brain. In other words, his profession required more mental work, rather than physical labor. His sleep needs, therefore, have revolved mainly around his brain rejuvenation, so he needed quite a lot of sleep when his brain was active. Joe was diligent in getting to bed at a reasonable hour and generally got his full eight or more hours. But right after his retirement, he took an extended vacation. He and his wife went on a few boat cruises, and the golf course was his hideaway. As a result, he found himself not sleeping as much as before. He went to bed a little later and became an early riser. Now this all stands to reason because his brain was not being used so much.

This is also true for someone who does heavy physical work, like Syd. He worked as a carpenter for a large construction company and did mainly physical labor. He had to climb scaffolds, lift heavy timber, and wield a heavy hammer. At the end of every day, he was very fatigued. In fact, he slept like a log most times.

When he retired, he found he had time on his hands. He took up golf with a buddy, puttered around the house, and did odd chores, but he suddenly found himself having difficulty staying asleep. He'd wake up at three in the morning and stare at the ceiling. Here again, his lifestyle change controlled his sleep. Not being so fatigued and not using his brain that much, his body didn't need as much rest. As a result, at least for the time being, he needed less sleep. However, that changed a few months later when he decided to do part-time construction and went to work with a friend who did small construction jobs. To his relief, his body went back to a healthy sleep cycle again.

The main point for me to emphasize here is that whenever you retire, or for that matter, make a change from doing heavy physical work to being more sedentary, you need to maintain active physical activity— as appropriate to your age and for at least as long as your health allows. Dramatic changes in your lifestyle can disrupt healthy sleep patterns. Also, your brain's sleep efficiency drops, so getting enough sleep may be more of a challenge than you realize.

Establishing healthy sleep patterns contributes to aging well. It will keep you healthy, enhance your immune system, sharpen your brain, and keep you safe. So whether you're a younger person with aging parents or an older person yourself, in addition to all the other sleep-enhancing principles I am laying out in this book, keep the following important points in mind for yourself and your elderly family members:

- Make sure you have any emerging health problem treated as soon as possible. Particularly be on the lookout for signs of sleep apnea and restless legs syndrome.
- Know the effects of all medications you are taking—both prescription and nonprescription, especially what they can do to your sleep. Often two medications taken by themselves may not be a problem, but when combined can cause a lot of reactions.

- Since the risk of depression increases with age, keep a lookout for it. As we age, our neurotransmitter systems decline in efficiency so depression can creep up unwittingly. Depression can disrupt sleep onset and sleep maintenance, as well as cause early morning waking. Depression can also cause severe fatigue, so a person may not want to get out of bed. There are effective medications for treating depression.
- Avoid big meals and limit fluids close to bedtime. If possible, switching to a midday main meal might also help. Also, the elderly need to particularly avoid caffeine, nicotine, and alcohol.
- Try to remain active and exercise daily, as appropriate for your age. Especially exercise your brain with jigsaw, crossword, or Sudoku puzzles, and keep it sharp by reading broadly and engaging in other mental activities. Remember this wise saying about the brain: You use it, or you lose it!

PART 3

OVERCOMING YOUR FAMILY'S SLEEP DEPRIVATION

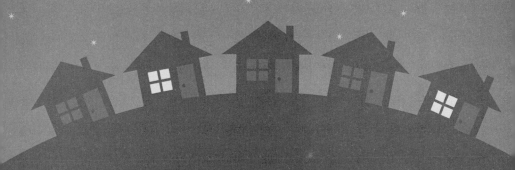

Helping Your Children Sleep Better

Sleep on, Baby, on the floor,
Tired of all the playing,
Sleep with smile the sweeter for,
That you dropped away in!
On your curls' full roundness stand
Golden lights serenely—
One cheek, pushed out by the hand,
Folds the dimple inly.
—ELIZABETH BARRETT BROWNING,
"SLEEPING AND WATCHING"

One of the encouraging signs that we might be attending more carefully to our children's sleep problems is the growing concern, now being widely expressed, over school starting times. Many now believe that the school day starts too early, reducing children's sleep time.

As children age, they undergo a biological change in their sleep pattern. Their readiness for sleep comes on later in the evening, as the child ages, and in older teenagers may even extend into the morning hours.[1] This is not just due to late-night TV and other distractions, though these things can aggravate the problem. It's the way we're designed. So, consider this: If your teen's biological sleep clock naturally pushes sleep onset too much later in the evening, then starting school early in the morning, which is a common practice in the U.S., might not be a good idea. To many researchers, forcing kids to start school early seems to work against nature. Teenagers staying up late and then needing to "sleep in" in the morning may not be a sign of rebellion or laziness. Their change in sleep habits may well be a natural part of growing up.

These findings have led many school systems to revise their school starting times, a move I heartily endorse. Since the natural tendency for teens is to only become sleepy later in the evening, if they are awakened early they are likely to be sleepy during the morning hours. The result is that many fall asleep in class during the first few hours of the day. To compensate for this, many school systems are exploring the effects of delaying starting times.

For instance, in 1997 the Minneapolis public school system changed its starting time from 7:15 AM to 8:40 AM, adding nearly one and a half hours to the students' sleep time. The change in start time proved effective. Results showed a marked improvement in attendance and learning, and a significant drop in student depression. Other schools have followed suit.

But there is another school-related problem often overlooked: homework. Problems here can be both the cause and the consequence of sleeplessness. No doubt, homework is essential to the learning process, but so also is sleep. It seems, however, that some educators place time spent doing homework above the need for sleep. We need to set limits on homework, but frankly not much research has been done here. Some studies suggest that "teenagers often sacrifice their sleep time when it comes to making choices about time management."[2] For instance, they might delay doing their homework earlier in the evening in order to engage in some recreational activity, but then find themselves running out of time and working on their homework late into the night.

So what can a parent do if you know that homework challenges are interfering with sleep? Obvious solutions, beyond the other sleep suggestions I offer in this chapter, include the following:

- Turn off the TV at night. Some teens fall asleep with the TV on, and some are so used to the noise they think they can't sleep without it. Obviously not true!

- Limit after-school activities. It's hard to do, but sometimes you just have to make hard choices!

- Prioritize those activities you want to keep. When running out of time, you need to know which must go first. This means striking a balance between making time for homework and time for sleep. Balance here will help your child's chances of getting into a great college. So know your priorities.

- Don't push challenging tasks on your child right before bedtime. It's hard to relax and get to sleep when your mind is stuck in some demanding mode (including video games). It takes a while to unwind, so maybe kids should tackle their hardest subject matter earlier.

- Turn off all cell phones. What's so important that it can't wait until morning? (However, some situations require an exception, such as having a parent who works at night and might need to stay in contact with his or her children.)

- Brainstorming ideas with the teacher may also be a good idea. For starters, it might be very helpful for your child's teacher to know that your child is struggling with homework, and that you are caught between a rock and a hard place, wanting your child to get enough sleep but also helping him or her to complete his or her homework assignments. This might also help reduce any tension your child may be feeling toward the teacher, and help the teacher get a better sense of how much homework is appropriate.

Obesity and Lack of Sleep

Not getting enough sleep can increase a child's risk of being overweight, according to a study by researchers at the Johns Hopkins School of Public Health. Their studies found that with each additional hour of sleep, the risk of being overweight drops by 9 percent.[3] Another study showed that babies and toddlers who sleep less than 12 hours daily are at greater risk for being overweight in pre-school. Television viewing heightened the effect. The children who slept the least and watched the most television had the greatest chance of becoming obese. It appears that while these two factors are quite independent, in combination they add health risks to children.[4]

What causes children to become obese, and why is it linked to lack of sleep? It appears that sleep impacts appetite, not just in children but also adults. Sleep-deprived people produce more ghrelin, a hormone that promotes the feeling of hunger, and less leptin, a hormone that signals fullness. So anything that robs you of sleep will increase your appetite. You will eat more and have difficulty knowing when you've eaten enough. The better you sleep, the fewer problems you will have eating and becoming overweight. A well-slept body will tell you when to stop eating. Isn't that amazing? So here we have a fantastic weight-reducing tool. Just get more sleep—but don't forget to exercise too!

Childhood Sleep Problems

There are important differences in sleep problems between children (under 12) and adolescents (13 and over) that you need to know about. Let me start with children, and then follow with adolescents.

Figure 6 summarizes childhood and teenage sleep disorders. Childhood sleep problems can be divided into two groups:

CHILDHOOD AND TEENAGE SLEEP DISORDERS		
Age	*Disorder*	*Intervention Strategy*
2 to 4 years:	Sleep onset difficulties	Predictable bedtime routine; system; firm limits; discipline
	Early waking difficulties	Earlier bedtime; identify causes (e.g., noise, light, etc.)
4 to 6 years:	Night terrors	Give bedtime reassurance; explore causes; counseling for fears
6 to 12 years:	Nocturnal enuresis	Avoid liquids after 3 p.m.; treat cause (e.g., bladder)
	Nocturnal encopresis	Void bowel before bedtime; main meal at lunch time
	Sleepwalking	Provide safe environment; alerting device; strategy for recovery
Adolescence:	Delayed sleep phase	Regular bedtime discipline
	Sleepwalking	Provide safe environment; alerting device; strategy for recovery
	Narcolepsy	Get professional help
	Sleep apnea	Get professional help

FIGURE 6: Childhood and Teenage Sleep Disorders

1. Physiological problems (like restless legs syndrome, sleep apnea, and narcolepsy). Many of these sleep disorders are more common in children than in adolescents.

2. Behavioral problems, where the child has a perfectly normal physiology. Examples are night terrors, sleepwalking, and enuresis (bed-wetting). Some children outgrow these disorders, but others may need professional help. (The term "behavioral problems" does not mean that

these problems are under the child's control. It is just a psychological term to indicate that these children are normal physically, so far as we can tell.)

Defining disordered sleep behavior in children is difficult because of important differences in sleep patterns at different stages of development. For example, it is not abnormal for a two-month-old to wake up frequently during the night. But if a two-year-old is doing it, it may be a problem. To make it even more difficult, families vary greatly in their tolerance of sleep habits. One family finds it problematic if a child isn't in bed by 9 PM, another only if it is past midnight.

Helping families resolve their children's sleep problems begins with a proper understanding of how children act differently at different ages. Then you can turn your attention to an equally challenging task: helping your children and teenagers get better and more sleep.

Let's begin with a sleep assessment questionnaire for your child.

Child Sleep Assessment Questionnaire

To help parents assess their child's sleep hygiene, I have put together the following assessment tool. Answer each question by circling a Yes or a No.

1. Does your child appear drowsy during the day for more than two days a week? Yes/No
2. Does your child show a reluctance to go to bed when you tell him or her to? Yes/No
3. Does your child have frequent wakings at night (several times each week)? Yes/No
4. Does your child go to bed before or after the following times: (answer only one)
   a. Under 10 years old: before 8 PM? Yes/No
   b. 11 to 13 years old: before 9 PM? Yes/No
   c. 14 to 16 years old: after 10 PM? Yes/No
   d. 17 or older: after 11 PM? Yes/No

5. Do you engage in a family activity of 30 minutes or longer at least three times a week just before they go to bed (such as board games, walks, talking, devotions, etc.)? Yes/No

6. If your child wakes up at night, does he or she have difficulty going back to sleep? Yes/No

7. Do you have to battle to get your child out of bed in the morning, at least three or more times a week? Yes/No

8. If your child wakes up at night, does he or she usually play quietly in bed? Yes/No

9. If your child is over six years of age, does he or she sleep in your bed with you more than once every two weeks? Yes/No

10. Are you concerned about your child's sleeping habits? Yes/No

SCORING: Count the number of times you circled Yes.

0 Yes's: This is ideal. Your child seems to be sleeping well.

If you have 1 or 2 Yes's: You may want to consider some minor changes to your child's sleep patterns.

3 to 5 Yes's: You need to start a program of sleep enhancement without delay.

6 or more Yes's: You may need to get some professional help.

If you are concerned about your child's sleep habits, regardless of your child's score here, get professional help right away.

Normal Sleep in Children

Let's begin with early-infant sleep. Infants (younger than six months) spend 50 percent of their sleep time in active dream sleep, compared with only 20 percent for adults. Until six months of age, therefore, children do not experience the same stages of sleep as adults do.

By six months, the infant's sleep patterns begin to resemble that of an adult's. After an initial "settling" period that typically takes 10 to 20 minutes, the infant drifts from stage 1 into stage 3 or 4 (all non-dream sleep). The first one-third of the night is mostly deep sleep, then it alternates between dream and non-dream sleep.

In newborns, the amount of sleep is divided fairly equally between night and day. Nighttime sleep gradually emerges over the first year, and daytime sleep gradually decreases over the first three years. By the age of four, most children no longer require a daytime nap. Nighttime sleep requirements also gradually decrease so that by adolescence, they are similar to the sleep needs of an adult.

It is estimated that up to 20 percent of young children are chronically sleep deprived.[5] When you consider the hectic schedules and busy lifestyles of families today, this is not surprising. When it comes to figuring out how much sleep your children need, you are better off just sticking with the recommended sleep times for different-aged children:

- For children aged 1 to 3 years old, 12 to 14 hours is recommended.
- For 3- to 6-year-olds, 11 to 12 hours.
- And for 7- to 12-year-olds, 10 to 11 hours.

Teenagers are more challenging. From 12 to 17 or even 18 years of age, they should be sleeping between 8.5 and 9.5 hours every night, or even longer. Here you might want to try the "incremental sleep adding" approach described in an earlier chapter, to see if you can determine the optimal sleep duration for your older teen. One hallmark of enough sleep is that irritability falls away, which is a sign of adequate sleep duration.

Bedtime Rituals for Children

One important factor in helping your children, especially young children, sleep well is by creating pleasant, memorable experiences at bedtime. One of the values of bedtime rituals is that they create a bond between children and parents. Many of my patients have told me stories of their bedtime rituals. I can't resist telling of my own bedtime rituals. They are precious memories.

As I was growing up in South Africa, my family wasn't well off. We lived in a part of town where houses were small, not to mention very hot in the summer. Because of the heat, many families, including mine, would sit on the front veranda in the early evening, savoring the fresh breezes. My father sat in a rocking chair, while my younger brother and I sat on the cool floor, leaning against the wall. He would tell us about his childhood escapades. He had been quite adventurous as a child, and while his escapades may have been a little exaggerated, they were true. Childhood in his day was very simple, so kids had to create their own excitement. To us, my father's escapades surpassed even those of the *Our Gang* kid's movies of my childhood. Plus, they had their effect: Sooner or later my brother and I fell asleep, and my father would carry us to bed.

And then there was my grandfather's bedtime ritual. My brother and I spent every school holiday with my wonderful grandparents. They lived out in the country on a small farm, and every evening, right after dark, we had a ritual: Water had to be pumped out of a closed well and up to a storage tank above the kitchen. The pump had a long handle and was mounted on a concrete slab over the well. It was all very simple. You moved the handle up and down, and it pumped the water. But even now, wonderful memories flood my mind as I recall listening to my grandfather tell us of his youthful adventures.

My brother and I would sit under the starry sky, close to where he sat working the pump. He had been a soldier in the British army during the Boer War from 1899 to 1902. Riding on horseback, he had covered thousands of miles in South Africa, in places filled with wild animals. And he *was* telling the truth; the lion-skin rugs on the floor gave credence to his escapades. When we would hear the telltale noise of water overflowing the tank, we knew it was bedtime.

But not only do bedtime rituals create enduring memories, they facilitate better sleep like nothing else. They provide a sense of security and love, and these must surely be the greatest sedatives of all.

So here are a few suggestions for creating a bedtime ritual for your children that will leave a lasting impression:

- Set clear bedtime rules and be consistent about when it is time for bed. Use a whistle or other signaling device to announce the start of their bedtime ritual. It can come to serve as an important conditioned cue for sleep.
- Set aside priority time for your children's ritual, say 20 or more minutes each evening, and be consistent yourself. In these days of stress and work pressures, parents need to give this time the highest priority.
- First, allow your children to tell you about their day or talk about whatever is on their minds. This helps to identify any bad experiences and gives you an opportunity to do some therapy. (Yes, moms and dads have to be therapists as well!)
- The actual ritual may vary depending on the child's age. For young children, you could start by reading a short story or Bible verse and explaining what it means, or tell them stories from your own childhood, as my father did when I was a child. Near the end, say something encouraging to each of your children. A great game you can create is to try and come up with something special each of your children did that day, and tell them how proud you are of them. Maybe Billy helped Mrs. Jones next door sweep her driveway; or Sarah, without being asked, volunteered to peel the potatoes. Find something your children did that day for which you are grateful and tell them so. Assure them that they are special. Rumor has it that the famous Dr. Phil used to whisper to his sons when they were small, "How do you suppose, out of all the little boys in the world, I got the best ones?"

- If your child is very young, rock him or her to sleep with a lullaby. You might let an older sibling rock the baby as well; this helps build family bonds. As your children get older, these rituals will take on a special significance to each of them.

- Remember, bedtime is separation time for children. It can be made easier by providing a transitional object, like a Teddy bear, doll, or blanket. Sometimes boys like to take something of their dad's to bed with them, like a scarf, handkerchief, hat, or book. It provides a symbolic bond that fosters security during the period of separation.

- Close with a short prayer. It helps to pray the same way each night so it becomes a regular experience. Not only does this teach them the value of prayer, but it will also help you bond with your children. Also, they will become better parents themselves one day for having had such a close encounter with your faith.

Adolescent Sleep Problems

The National Institutes of Health (NIH) have identified adolescents and young adults (ages 12 to 25 years) as a population at high risk for sleep problems based on "evidence that the prevalence of problem sleepiness is high and increasing in these gaps with particularly serious consequences."[6] NIH further warns that urgent steps need to be taken to reduce the risks associated with sleep deprivation in our teens and young adults. And they mean *urgent*.

There are many factors that can negatively impact adolescent sleep in our modern world. An important study conducted recently by Columbia University looked at the effect that television watching had on teenagers. They found that adolescents who watched three hours or more of television per day had a significantly elevated risk for sleep problems by early adulthood—regardless of age, gender, or home factors.[7]

Teenagers who reduced television watching by one or more hours a day experienced a significant drop in their risk for sleep problems.

Every parent knows that adolescents don't sleep like the rest of us. Adolescent sleep is characterized by lack of consistency, irregular sleep schedules, daytime sleepiness, and elevated risk for sleep disturbances. But when paired together, insomnia, nightmares, and sleep insufficiency are commonly associated with elevated risk for suicide in depressed teenagers.[8] So if your teenager is depressed, fostering better sleep habits is one positive protection you can give him or her. And don't forget that modeling good sleep habits can go a long way toward encouraging your teens to do the same.

To help parents assess their adolescents' sleep hygiene, I have put together two questionnaires. The first assesses your teen's general level of sleepiness, while the second explores your teen's sleep habits. The first is worded so your teenager can take it directly, or you can answer it on behalf of your teen if you believe you know what he or she is experiencing. The second is worded so a parent can answer the questions. Be warned: The issues here can easily be fudged by the teenager.

Adolescent Sleep Assessment Questionnaire

Answer each question by circling a Yes or a No.

1. Do you fall asleep during morning classes several times a month? Yes/No
2. Do you fall asleep during the last class of the day? Yes/No
3. Do you feel tired most of the day at school for a couple of days each week? Yes/No
4. Do you go to bed after 10:30 PM during the school week? Yes/No
5. Is it difficult for you to intentionally exercise regularly (play sports, etc.)? Yes/No

6. Is it often difficult for you to get up for school in the morning?
    Yes/No

7. Do you often have arguments with other members of your
    family? Yes/No

8. Do you fall asleep easily whenever you ride in a car for longer
    than five minutes? Yes/No

9. Do you have to have music playing (headphones, iPod, etc.) to
    fall asleep? Yes/No

10. Do you feel sleepy when you do your homework a lot of the
    time? Yes/No

SCORING: Count the number of times you circled Yes. Ideally,
you should have no Yes's.

0 to 1 Yes's: You seem to be sleeping enough.

2 to 4 Yes's: You may need to get more sleep.

Over 4 Yes's: You are seriously sleep deprived and need to give the
highest priority to getting more sleep.

In addition to assessing your teenager's sleepiness, it is also important that you pay attention to your teen's sleeping habits. Bad sleep
habits, when established in adolescence, will almost certainly become a
lifetime bad habit with serious health consequences.

Teen Sleep Habit
Checklist

Here is a checklist to help you identify your teenager's sleep habits. Each
question relates to an important aspect of your teen's habits. From what
you have already read, you should be able to evaluate these habits and
determine where you need to focus your attention.

Circle a Yes or a No for your teenager. The more Yes answers
your teenager has, the greater the likelihood that he or she has a sleep
problem.

1. Has your teenager's sleep problem lasted for longer than one year? Yes/No
2. Has your teenager's sleep problem gotten worse recently? Yes/No
3. Is your teenager experiencing a lot of stress in school or work? Yes/No
4. Is your teenager experiencing stress in relationships? Yes/No
5. Does your teenager share a bedroom with a sibling or other person? Yes/No
6. Does your teenager resist going to bed when told to? Yes/No
7. Does your teenager wake up easily and frequently during the night? Yes/No
8. Does your teenager sleep for less than eight hours a night? Yes/No
9. Does your teenager usually "crash" on weekends and sleep late and long? Yes/No
10. Does your teenager watch TV or videos in bed before going to sleep? Yes/No
11. Does your teenager play video or Internet games before going to sleep? Yes/No
12. Does your teenager avoid hobbies, preferring TV or Internet activities? Yes/No
13. Has your teenager ever had to take sleep medication for more than a month's time? Yes/No
14. Is your teenager tardy in getting to school more than one day a month? Yes/No

This checklist covers the most common sleep disrupters in a teen's life. All the Yes answers point you to where changes need to be made.

How Much Sleep Does Your Teen Need?

As a general rule, adolescents need somewhere between 8.5 hours and 9.5 hours of sleep on a regular basis.[9] However, many experts now believe that teenagers need more sleep than this, and certainly more than an adult because of the extensive learning tasks that abound at this stage of development.

I mentioned earlier that an adolescent's sleep pattern undergoes a "phase delay" during this stage of life. That is, in the late teen years there is a natural tendency toward only feeling tired enough to go to bed much later in the evening. No one knows the reason for this, but this is why teenagers want to stay up later and find it more difficult to get to bed earlier. Parents may need to adjust their teen's morning routine to allow for some extra sleep time, because the delayed tiredness of the night before pushes wakefulness back as well. An example would be delaying the start of school till later or ensuring that the teen doesn't have to get up early because other family members have to get up early.

That teens often want more sleep over the weekend is not a bad thing. As you will see when I discuss our "sleep bank" in a later chapter, this is one way teenagers can make up for sleep lost during the week.

What Can You Do to Help Your Teen?

Since teens need 8.5 to 9 hours of sleep a night (minimum), you don't need to be a math whiz to figure out that if they wake up for school at 6 AM, they must go to bed by 9 PM to reach the nine-hour mark. Many teens have trouble falling asleep this early since they are still "wired" from their MP3 players and computer games. It's not because they don't want to sleep. It's because their brains have been stimulated late into the evening and aren't ready for sleep.

And even when the teenager goes to bed early, falling asleep is another challenge. I hear from many teenagers that they can only go to sleep listening to music. The problem is that modern teen music is usually loud and upbeat—designed to keep you awake, not put you to sleep.

While the most common cause of teenage insomnia is stress, other things can lead to insomnia as well, including physical discomfort (the stuffy nose of a cold or the pain of a headache), emotional troubles (like family problems or relationship difficulties), and even an uncomfortable sleeping environment (a room that's too hot, cold, or noisy).

If your teen is having sleep problems, try as many of the following solutions as possible:

- By whatever means possible, try to enforce regular bedtime hours. Nothing is more important to the brain's sleep/wake mechanisms than the regular resetting of the sleep clock. I have convinced some of my teenage grandchildren to get to bed earlier by merely challenging them to sleep one hour longer every night for one week, and see for themselves the difference it makes.

- Get your teen to bed as early as possible—according to his or her age. "Early to bed and early to rise" is wise counsel.

- If your teen wants to listen to music when going to sleep, make sure it is relaxing music. Some find the sound of "white noise" or nature, such as the ocean or forest, to be soothing for sleep. Devices are available to produce these sounds.

- Avoid bedtime snacks, particularly grains and sugars. These will raise your teen's blood-sugar level and inhibit sleep. Later, when the blood-sugar level drops too low (hypoglycemia), he or she might wake up and not be able to fall back asleep again.

• Your child/teen *must* sleep in complete darkness or as close to it as possible. A low-level night-light, kept out of direct view, might be okay. However, even the tiniest bit of light can disrupt the circadian rhythm and the production of melatonin.

• Take the TV out of the bedroom. The temptation is too great. Watching TV is too stimulating to the brain, and your teen will take longer to fall asleep. Also, many teens don't have the self-discipline to regulate their TV watching.

• Avoid using loud alarm clocks to wake up your teen. The interruption of deep sleep by a loud alarm, especially during the dreaming stage, is very stress producing. It causes quite a surge of adrenaline. And here parents have a challenge. If you are already up and about, then you might find it better to gently wake your teen yourself (for instance, by being noisy, or, if necessary, knocking on his or her door). Alternatively, new types of alarm clocks are now available that start soft, then increase in sound until they break down your resistance. This might make waking up a teen less stressful to you.

• Try to expose your teen to sunlight as early as possible after he or she gets up. This helps to turn off melatonin and sleepiness. Walking to school is better than driving him or her—if this is possible.

• Avoid caffeine after 3 PM. This includes energy drinks, sodas, chocolate, and so on. Caffeine is not metabolized efficiently in teens, and therefore they can feel the effects long after consuming it. Also, any medications that have caffeine in them should be avoided in the early evening.

• Lose weight. If your teen is overweight, there will be an increased risk of sleep apnea and diabetes. Your child may also develop acid reflux—a surge of gastric juices up the esophagus when he or she lies down to go to sleep. If so, try raising the head of the bed a few inches by placing wood blocks under the headboard. Also, if you suspect your teen has these problems, discuss them with his or her doctor.

• Encourage taking a hot bath or shower before going to bed. A pleasant "going to bed" ritual like this can improve sleep onset in all of us.

Closing

There is no doubt in my mind that the greatest sleep challenge facing us today as parents is to confront the rapidly declining sleep patterns in our children. Facing an onslaught of stimulating gadgets outside of school, excitement is now a 24/7 (and you can add 365 days a year) experience. Everything from video and Internet games, online social networks, and MP3 players—you name it—they spell E-X-C-I-T-E-M-E-N-T of the sort that can keep children awake.

I agree with Dennis Prager, a well-known sociologist and syndicated radio show host, who says that young people today have more excitement available to them than any generation in history.[10] He also believes that excitement has become our most dangerous drug today, robbing our children and teens of the happiness they so much deserve. I would add, however, that the sleep it robs them of is the main cause of the diminished happiness and contentment and, at times, increased boredom that we see in the world of youth today.

Sleep and Your Marriage

Marriage is an alliance entered into
by a man who can't sleep with the window shut,
and a woman who can't sleep with the window open.
—GEORGE BERNARD SHAW

Laugh and the world laughs with you; snore and you sleep alone.
—ANTHONY BURGESS

Believe it or not, sleep can make or break a marriage. I'm serious! While it's easy to see how bad marriages can cause sleep problems and might then end in divorce, it is equally important to keep the reverse in mind. Sleep deprivation can alter the dynamics of a marriage to such an extent that it cannot survive. And the reasons are very clear. Sleep deprivation makes you cranky, irritable, angry, and unhappy. How could you possibly communicate, listen, or empathize? You become critical and judgmental, even depressed, and these all have an effect on the marital relationship.

My wife and I have had our sleep-deprived moments. I am just fortunate that my wife, early in our marriage, recognized the importance of sleep. She needed more sleep than I did and was the one who insisted we invest in earplugs, good mattresses and pillows, and healthful sleeping habits. I have no doubt that improving our sleep helped us through difficult times by keeping all those nasty, sleep-deprived behaviors and emotions at bay.

And taking care of your marriage is important. Building a happy marriage does not come about by chance. It takes careful attention to detail, and one of the details is sleep.

Couples spend one-third of their lives sleeping together, so sleep is bound to have an impact on marriage. And this isn't just my opinion. Two recent studies reported in the *New York Times* found that if you improve your sleep, you improve your marriage.[1]

Also, women who are married appear to sleep better than women who have never married or who have lost a partner, according to an eight-year study.[2] But it's a two-way street. They also found that marital happiness lowers the risk of sleep problems, while marital strife heightens it.

The truth is that no two people are perfectly compatible—in any way or form—and this applies to how we sleep as well. I have always been cynical about the notion that there is a "perfect match" out there somewhere. That if only you could find him or her, you could guarantee a happy marriage. I believe that success at marriage is not about "finding" the right partner; it's about "becoming" the right partner. When we marry, we not only bring different personalities, backgrounds, habits, and attitudes to the relationship, we also bring a host of other differences. That's the beauty of it all! No matter how much we thought we were compatible, the day we marry is the start of a profound call to change. And only partners willing to make changes can survive.

Another way of saying this is that incompatibility is the given, not the exception. We will have different sleep needs and habits from the start. How can they not be different, given that we have different genes, differ in gender, and grew up in different families? What this means is that every marriage will require some re-ordering in many areas, including in the sleep domain. Like it or not, our sleep habits will have to change and become synchronized to some extent. Either that or live in separate homes! The bonus is, of course, a happier marriage. I wonder at times whether God thought up marriage as a sort of inbuilt psychotherapy? It sure feels like it at times.

Sleep's Impact on Marriage

Let's examine sleep's impact on marriage, or vice versa, a little deeper. A National Sleep Foundation survey found the following:[3]

- Twelve percent of married couples sleep alone—that is, they have chosen to sleep in separate bedrooms. This could be that they can get better sleep this way, or because one of the partners is a "sleep disrupter." Sleeping in your own bed without a partner rocking and rolling, wheezing and whistling, sneezing and snoring, can improve sleep habits.

- Good sleep and marital satisfaction are related. This confirms my opening statements. Marriages where one or both of the partners have insomnia, and therefore daytime sleepiness, report a lower level of marital satisfaction. But what is cause and effect here? Does bad sleep make you unhappy, or does a bad marriage cause you to be sleepless? Possibly both. All we know is that there is a clear link between marital happiness and good sleep.

- Twelve percent of married couples report sleeping with a child—and this adds sleep disruptions. Eighty-one percent of the couples who allow a child to sleep with them report having a sleep problem. Also, research indicates that co-sleeping with a baby raises the risk of sudden infant death syndrome.[4]

- Snoring is a common complaint—and the source of a lot of sleep disruption. There are many causes of snoring that I covered earlier in the book. But the most serious cause, sleep apnea, should be remedied as early as possible. Keep in mind that it can occur at any age.

- With disturbed sleep comes a drop in sexual libido. On the other hand, a healthy sex life can do wonders for sleep—so there is a two-way benefit here. For men, sex is usually a form of tranquilizer. It offers a soothing sleep inducer. For women, it is more often a stimulant and may delay sleep onset for a while. However, let me hasten to add that couples and individuals differ widely here, so one should not generalize.

It is clear from the National Sleep Foundation's survey mentioned earlier that sleeplessness can drive you apart, and that there are a number of sleep issues every married couple must face.

Imagine the following scenario: Cindy and Robert have been married now for two and a half years. They have a 12-month-old baby just starting to teethe and Robert is in a major transition at work, taking on new responsibilities that require him to be "on the ball" every minute of the day. They have a queen-sized bed that seemed sufficient when they first married, but it's getting cramped. Cindy gets up several times during most nights to check on their baby and often throws off the covers in frustration as she stumbles in a daze to the nursery. When she gets back into bed, she has to shove Robert to get him to roll back to his side and stop his snoring so she can get back to sleep. And as soon as she falls asleep again, Robert's snoring explodes and wakes her up. Frustrated, she grabs her pillow, yanks the blanket off Robert, and storms bleary-eyed into their living room to sleep another night on the couch. This is not what they'd expected in marriage. They had expected that sleep would be a unifier and that each evening they would happily drift off in each other's arms.

Every night, countless couples battle sleep issues like this. So let's look at some ways in which couples can learn to sleep peacefully. Newlyweds often don't discover that they have a problem until after the honeymoon stage of the marriage. Pre-marital counseling rarely addresses the issue of sleep.

Simple Solutions to Complex Problems

What is somewhat distressing to me, as I reflect on many of the couples with marital problems I have counseled, is how easily most of their sleep conflicts can be rectified if only they took the trouble. Couples with seemingly insurmountable sleep problems often settle into a state of "learned helplessness," believing that their differences in sleep patterns can't be fixed. Learned helplessness is a state of mind in which you believe that you are helpless to change something that is bothering you, so you settle into believing you have no control. As a result, you stay passive in the face of unpleasant, or even damaging, circumstances.

To illustrate, let me tell you about Mary and Michael. Empty nesters (with two married sons now living on their own) in the 26th year of marriage, they now have the whole house to themselves. However, every night before going to bed they both use the master bathroom for their nightly routines, which they prefer to do in private. Michael is an accountant and Mary a schoolteacher, so both live busy lives and are pretty exhausted by bedtime. Sleep is a high priority for both of them, so there is no problem there. But getting to bed always leads to an argument. Mostly they argue over the use of the bathroom, and invariably become so angered with each other that it prevents them from falling asleep peacefully. By the time they got up the courage to seek help, they had begun considering a separation.

What was it about the bedtime bathroom ritual that enraged them? Each accused the other of taking too much time. And each had a plausible explanation for why he or she had to take so much time to get ready for bed.

The battle for the bathroom starts just after finishing their evening duties. Mary often has some schoolwork to prepare, while Michael has to sort out his paperwork for the next day. As bedtime nears, one or the other opens up the conversation with, "Is it okay if I use the bathroom first?" "Well, I want to take a bath and you'll use up all the hot water." "But you always take such a long time that I'm too tired to have a bath when it comes to my turn. It's better if I go first."

Sometimes the "first come, first served" rule dominates. One or the other tries to sneak off quietly when the other isn't looking, so as to get in first. Sometimes there is a mad rush, with one claiming an emergency that urgently needs attention, and then claiming the bathroom for the rest of the ablutions. Sometimes they would toss a coin—until Mary discovered that Michael was using a trick quarter he had acquired from a magic shop during a conference visit to Las Vegas. Yes, you guessed it. It had two heads—or tails; I can't remember which! This was the straw that broke the camel's back and they sought help.

I listened to both sides of the story, carefully and empathically. But to be honest, I kept imagining a Laurel and Hardy comedy routine. But to Mary and Michael this was serious stuff. Then a simple question popped into my mind. Even as I asked it, though, I felt quite stupid, as if I were becoming part of Laurel and Hardy's battle over a bathroom. "How many bathrooms do you have?" Stunned silence.

They looked at each other, then back at me. "Why is that important? We're talking about a major conflict here, not about how many bathrooms we have," Michael said. I remained silent—often the best form of therapy. The room was quiet for a while. Then finally, Mary responded with: "We have two bathrooms. One is ours, and the other is the boys'. We've always kept it as it was when they lived at home. We want them to feel that it is still their home when they come to stay over." The answer was staring us in the face, but they still couldn't see it. So I had to take the prompting step further.

"But your boys don't live at home with you anymore, do they, and only come to stay over once in a while?" The truth is that one of their sons lived in the same neighborhood, and their other son lived across town, and neither ever came to "stay over." Slowly, the point I was trying to make sank in. It was close. For a moment it looked as if it wasn't going to get to first base, let alone past it. "Yes . . . but when they want to come and visit, it's there for them to use," Mary said. Another silent pause as the prospect of a solution dawned. Then a slow, feeble response from Michael: "But it's still their bathroom." He wasn't going to give up without a fight.

"What would it take to remodel the boys' bathroom so that it no longer looks and feels like their bathroom? Then one of you could claim it as your bathroom, and if and when one of the boys comes to visit, it can be available for him."

Mary was the first to smile. "Okay, but Michael will have to move to the other bathroom—not me."

"I suppose I could," Michael said. After a pause he continued, "Why didn't we think of this?" When they left, though, you could still hear him muttering, "But it is really the boys' bathroom, isn't it?"

Turns out that after a fresh coat of paint, some window frosting, new curtains, and a radio for the bathroom, Michael, Mary told me, was "grinning like a possum eating persimmons" as he took possession of it as his own, boys-only, no-intruders-allowed space. Problem fixed. No more battles from then on, and no more sleep problems either.

Now I realize that not all sleep disruptions are so easily resolved. And you might be thinking, as I did, that in this case the answer was obvious. But how often do we allow something seemingly trivial to cause a wedge between us and our spouses? I know it's happened in my marriage and probably has in yours, too. Couples soon enough discover that sleep-related conflicts are many: which side of the bed is preferred, what time to go to bed, when to get up, where to put the dresser, and on and on. Many couples believe that their differences are cast in concrete and nothing can be done to change them. That's just not true. So let's consider some common problems and their possible solutions.

Marriage and Your Bed

Another, more obvious, marital conflict revolves around the bed. It certainly was a major issue for my wife and me. When we got married, we were in South Africa where a Dutch-Reformed theology prevailed. When you marry, you have to sleep in the same bed as your spouse. No arguments. It was expected. Sleeping apart, many feared, was a sign that your marriage is in trouble.

But the idea of a one-bed marriage is really just a myth. If you choose to always sleep in the same bed, then God bless your marriage. But there is no law, biblical or otherwise, that says couples must sleep together in one bed, so don't let this belief control your marriage. Take my own marriage, for example. I was the one who insisted from the start that ours was to be a one-bed marriage. I'd heard of couples who slept in two beds, and a part of me kept wondering if they were in trouble. For me, however, it was to be one bed.

And for the first few months, it was wonderful. Our bed was certainly not king-sized when we married many years ago. In fact, we had never seen, nor even heard of, king-sized beds. One probably wouldn't have fit into our small bedroom anyway. We slept like spoons neatly packed together, and quickly learned the art of turning in tandem. The problem was that when one turned, the other had to wake up to turn also.

To be honest, it wasn't all that bad during the early stage of our marriage. You certainly couldn't sustain a pout for long when you were so close. And I loved the closeness, the warmth, the intimacy, the shared experience, the tender moments before falling asleep. But reality caught up with us after our first child was born. It then became impossible for both of us to get enough sleep when one of us had to get up many times a night to feed the baby or change the baby's diaper.

Needless to say, this made us grumpy and disagreeable. Every time my wife turned over or got up, I had to turn also. Every time she coughed, I almost coughed too. It was "stereo sleeping," never out of sync but seldom beneficial to either of us. For quite a few years we believed that this "slumber closeness" was essential to a happy marriage.

Then, heaven blessed us. After having three children, I built a large home for us. And queen-sized beds arrived. We splurged and recovered a bit of heaven. It was pure luxury to not have to turn in sync just to stay in bed!

Soon after, we moved to the U.S., and the first bit of furniture we bought was a king-sized bed. But it wasn't long before we realized that even king-sized beds could still be disruptive to sleep. The bed rocks and rolls no matter how big it is. So finally, my wife and I decided that for the sake of our sanity (and our marriage) it was imperative that we each get a good night's sleep. We bit the bullet and invested in two twin beds. But we park them right next to each other (a few inches apart) so we can still hold hands when we go to sleep. It immediately, and effectively, unlinked our sleep movements. Now I can toss and turn to my heart's content. And we haven't lost an ounce of intimacy!

However, bed manufacturers are becoming more and more sophisticated in designing beds and mattresses, and it may be worth your while to do a little research here and see if you can find a bed that suits your need. Beds are available with remotes that can control each side of the bed. Even mattresses are being designed in such a way that if one person moves around, the other side of the bed never moves. So these are accessible possibilities worth exploring.

Two Major Pre-Sleep Destroyers

My middle daughter, Dr. Sharon (Hart) May, is a marriage and family therapist. Most of her therapy is conducted in intensive sessions where couples work all day for several days trying to repair their damaged relationships. It is a very effective form of marital therapy. I was recently discussing with her the role sleep plays in building a successful marriage, and she told me that from her experience with many couples, she's noticed two major "sleep destroyers" that can contribute to marital problems. The first is a couple's failure to resolve arguments at bedtime. The second is a couple's failure to synchronize their sleep patterns—time and length. Let's take a look at each of these.

Unresolved Arguments Before Bedtime

Bill and Judy go to bed at their usual time. As they settle down, Bill raises the hot topic of deciding where they will spend their summer holiday, desiring a brief discussion so that it can be resolved before going to sleep. He wants them, including their two teenage sons, to go to Michigan where his parents have a lakeside family cabin. But Judy would prefer Hawaii, her favorite vacation place. The weather is warm there, and the boys are old enough to swim. Besides, they haven't been back there since their honeymoon so many years ago. Bill accuses Judy of not liking his mother. Judy accuses Bill of being a cheapskate and not wanting to spend the extra money for a hotel in Hawaii. The argument escalates—and not at a good time either, because anger inevitably causes an adrenaline surge that, in turn, turns off the body's need for sleep. Prebedtime arguments are seldom resolved before bedtime, and they always disrupt sleep.

As expected, they both lie steaming mad in bed. Bill is the withdrawer, so he turns over and, with his back to Judy, gives her the "silent treatment." Judy is the pursuer, so she pleads with him for some resolution before they go to sleep. He counters that he has to get up early for work, ". . . so let's just drop the topic!"

According to my daughter's records over the past eight years, 80 percent of wives cannot get to sleep after an argument. They need to talk a problem through and arrive at some resolution before they can turn it off. On the other hand, 80 percent of husbands are incapable of talking through a difference without getting angry and withdrawing. True, these couples were in therapy because they had additional problems, but it's not so different for those couples not in therapy.

Judy thinks, *He just doesn't love me anymore.* Bill thinks, *She doesn't care about what I want.* She sobs silently, tears soaking her pillow. He sulks himself into a morose three-day moodiness—the national standard for a male sulk! Sleep can't take this sort of conflict, so it withdraws also.

There are three principles that you need to follow to prevent arguments at bedtime from disrupting your sleep, and possibly your marriage:

1. Never open up a topic that is likely to be contentious just before you go to bed. Especially avoid all potential arguments once you are in bed. This is not the time to solve personal or schedule problems.

2. If you find yourself in an argument or heated discussion about any topic, call a truce as soon as possible. Husbands, turn to your wife and tell her you love her, that you both need your rest, and that you need more time to work through the issue, "so let's discuss it in the morning when we are fresh and rested." Wives, understand that talking things through when both parties are rested usually ends with better results.

3. If you do not have good argument skills—and by this I mean knowing how to argue in a healthy way—then I recommend you read my daughter's book *How to Argue So Your Spouse Will Listen.*[5] Resolving arguments is a skill you can learn.

Failure to Synchronize Sleep Patterns

This is the second most common sleep destroyer in marriage. No matter how compatible a couple you might think you are when you are dating, reality is that you are as different in your sleep patterns as chalk is from cheese. Your daily body rhythms are going to be different, as will your pre-sleep rituals. For one thing, males invariably have a different circadian rhythm than females. Their body clocks are saying "awake" when their partner's clock is saying "sleep."

Here is a typical scenario. Alan is a TV addict. He's hooked on late-night talk shows and any game whatsoever—baseball, basketball, wrestling, bowling—you name it, he goes for it, as long as it is on late-night TV! He is what is popularly known as a "night person." This means he likes to go to bed late. He also likes to get up late, and this has become a problem as well. He invariably starts his day sluggishly. Not till he's had two java fixes at the local coffee shop can he even keep his head upright and his eyelids open. Around midday he begins to feel energetic. Got the picture?

Helen, on the other hand, is a "morning person." She likes to get to bed early and get up early. Early morning is her best and most productive time. She comes alive when the sun rises; loves to take an early morning walk; and launches the day like a rocket going to the moon! But by early evening she comes back to earth all fizzled out. If she had her way she'd gladly go to bed at sunset.

Now who is right? Neither, of course. This out-of-step sleep pattern is called a "sleep rhythm difference" (night persons living with morning persons—if having a label for it offers any consolation). If you have this rhythm difference in your marriage, you need to address the following issues:

- Sleeping together—and I mean at the same time, not just in the same bed—is all about compromise. As a couple you need to come to some mutually acceptable sleep plan. Discuss how you can overlap your rhythm differences. What is extremely important here is not to believe the myth that so-called morning and evening persons are this way because they were born this way, and cannot change. There is no gene that determines how you sleep—it is pure habit. A husband could have learned his rhythm pattern from his father, or a wife from her mother, but it is neither genetic nor inherent. These are habits that are learned and can be changed. Yes, it may be difficult to unlearn them, but not impossible.

Remember, we have to shift our sleep/wake times up or down by an hour twice a year to accommodate daylight savings time. So if we can change an hour twice a year, why can't we shift our sleep times longer and create a happier marriage as well? Be willing to give a little so you can take a little.

- Try to find a mutually enjoyable nighttime ritual for you both to engage in before going to bed—something you can do together, even if one of you goes to bed before the other. It is this shared time together that you miss out on if you go to bed at different times. You could play a card game, take a walk, or watch something on TV you have recorded. For instance, if there is something on TV late at night that I would love to watch, I program my storage device, like TiVo, to save it for me so that my wife and I can watch it together at a more convenient time. Problem solved!

- If you and your spouse are at opposite ends of the sleep rhythm, then both of you should begin to gradually shift your pattern to a healthy center position. But change it slowly. It adapts to small changes better and easier than it does to large changes. So, wife, go to bed a little later and get up a little later. Husband, go to bed a little earlier and get up a little earlier—or vice versa!

Make Compromises

If you are having trouble sleeping in the same bed together because you have differing sleep patterns, try compromising and meeting somewhere in the middle. More often than not, one of you likes to go to sleep much later than the other. So split the difference. You go to bed an hour earlier and your spouse can go to bed an hour later. After a while you will both learn how to adapt to the change. The same with getting up. Try finding a compromise on bedtimes.

One of the more positive values in sleeping together is that it increases your sense of intimacy. It also lowers your stress and may help prevent arguments. Compromising needs to be the game plan for many of the following differences we bring to marriage:

- Who gets which side of the bed?
- What sleep positions do we use?
- When do we have sex?
- Temperature of the room?
- To cuddle or not to cuddle before sleeping?
- How to toss or turn?
- Degree of quietness?
- The size of the bed?
- The firmness of the bed?
- Who controls the heat blanket thermostat?
- Having a window open or closed?
- Sleeping with children or pets?
- Number of blankets?

Whether you are newlyweds or have been married for years, taking a look at these questions together can help you proactively move toward having healthful sleeping habits in your home.

Give Love Gifts

Early in our marriage, my wife, Kathleen, and I made a discovery. Even though we were closely attached, emotionally, spiritually, and in many other ways, we were struggling in our relationship because we seemed to be so different in what we wanted to do. Things I liked doing, she didn't. Things she liked doing, I didn't.

I learned how to fly an airplane when we still lived in South Africa, but she refused to fly with me. "It's too dangerous," she said. When we moved to the U.S. I bought a used sailboat and turned to sailing. One of my sons-in-law loved sailing, so we quickly became competent sailors on the Pacific Ocean. Then I invited my wife to come sailing with us. But apparently her gastric system didn't care for rocking and rolling on the big sea, so that was the end of our sailing together.

I longed for something we could do together. To cut a long story short, not long after immigrating to the U.S. I received an invitation to give some lectures at a seminary in Australia. I rushed home to share the excitement with my wife and suggested she go with me. But she declined, saying she doesn't handle jetlag well. I was most disappointed—and showed it! Then a few days later, to my surprise, she said the following while lying in bed: "Sweetheart, you know that traveling internationally is not my favorite thing, but I can sense how much you want me to go with you. What I will do is give you a 'love gift' this time. I'll go with you."

And thus was born a strategy we have used for many years as a way of overcoming our differences. Whenever we find ourselves differing in what we want to do, we consider whether or not to give each other a love gift. A love gift could be me saying, "I want more than anything for you to go with me, but my love gift to you is my blessing to stay home." Love gifts can also apply to the differences in our sleeping patterns. A love gift is doing something that you ordinarily wouldn't want to do.

But because you love each other so much, you sacrifice your own need to fulfill the need of your partner.

It's a compromise with a difference—you quickly learn that a love gift builds the appreciation of your partner. Over the years we have developed a few "rules" for giving love gifts. For one thing, you cannot give a love gift and then gripe about not liking it afterward. Also, you cannot ask for a love gift. It must be freely given without invitation or coercion, or else it is not a gift. You cannot "trade" love gifts, like, "Honey, last month I went to that restaurant you like, so would you please go to the game with me on Saturday?" Also, there can be no retaliation if no gift is offered. It has to be a "gift" in every sense of the word. If you don't get one, be gracious and loving nevertheless.

When it comes to sleeping together, the experience will be easier if you develop your skills at giving love gifts. What might this look like?

Karen and John had been married a little more than a year and were frustrated by their lack of agreement when it came to sleeping. Karen felt that it was nice to fall asleep in each other's arms. John wanted to make his wife happy, but just couldn't sleep comfortably that way. This became a source of stress; every night they knew that one or both of them would end up with hurt feelings. Karen felt unloved and disappointed whenever John turned his back to her to go to sleep. John felt frustrated that Karen couldn't let it go and let him get some sleep. Sound petty? As we've established, sometimes the smallest issues in a marriage can result in stress.

In this case, it was Karen's love gift to John that allowed him to sleep how he was most comfortable, without worrying that she would be resentful or keep bringing it up.

Take a moment to consider in what areas you and your spouse might need to exchange love gifts. "Love gifting" has become a way of life for my wife and me. It helps overcome our differences and builds a special love because it pleases our partner. And guess what? The gift you give your partner becomes a blessing to yourself as a bonus.

Managing Your Family's "Sleep Bank"

Now I lay me down to sleep,
I pray the Lord my soul to keep;
When in the morning light I wake,
Teach me the path of love to take.
—A MODERN VERSION OF A CLASSIC CHILD'S PRAYER

In 1995, the National Commission on Sleep Disorders Research, established by President Clinton, published a groundbreaking report entitled "Wake Up America."[1] The commission, drawn from many experts around the world, had evaluated the status of insomnia and other sleep disorders in the U.S. and reported that insomnia was both prevalent and costly. It also predicted that the issue of insomnia would continue to rise in the years ahead. Now we are more than 15 years further down this road, and exactly as predicted, it has gotten worse.

I remember when the call for the establishment of a sleep commission went out. I was on a speaking tour of Australia at the time and was surprisingly impressed to discover that Australia was way ahead of the U.S. in this matter. For instance, wherever I went I saw large signs across freeways warning drivers to "BEWARE MICROSLEEPS." You couldn't miss them. The idea of "microsleeps" was then quite foreign to the U.S. public, and still is to some extent. But every Australian I met knew what it meant.

So what is a microsleep? It is what happens when you are sleep deprived and tired, causing you to fall asleep easily—perhaps for only a fraction of a second or a few seconds—and then you wake up without realizing that you've been out of it. Long-distance drivers are particularly at risk. When an exhausted driver dozes for just a few seconds— that's long enough to cause a catastrophe on the freeway. You may not have even closed your eyes. But you were actually asleep!

The findings of the president's commission on sleep were most illuminating and taught me a number of lessons about sleep. My reason for mentioning it here is that what follows comes largely out of one of the commission's recommendations for fixing our sleep problem.

How's Your "Sleep Bank"?

You may not realize it, but just as you have a money bank account, you also have a sleep bank account. This is how the commission suggested we think about sleep. I have found the bank metaphor to be extremely helpful, because it suggests many appropriate analogies.

In introducing this new way of thinking about sleep, the commission summarized the following relevant points to keep in mind:

- We make deposits when we sleep, and we make withdrawals when we are awake. It's better to have a positive sleep balance in this account and not a negative one—that is, to be in the black with a surplus of accumulated sleep.
- Not getting enough sleep means you could be "overdrawn" at the sleep bank—that is, in the red with a deficiency of accumulated sleep.
- As with all overdrafts, there is a penalty to be paid for being overdrawn. In the case of your sleep bank, an overdraft (sleep deprivation) can seriously affect your well-being, your health,

and even your longevity. The penalty can be emotional, physical, or spiritual.

• If you are excessively overdrawn at your sleep bank, your risk for serious stress and illnesses goes up because your immune system is compromised,[2] and emotional well-being comes down because of disrupted brain function, such as an increase in anxiety due to stress.[3]

• To reduce these consequences you need to keep your sleep account in the black, and current overdrafts should be cancelled by depositing "make-up" sleep as soon as possible.

• We can add to our sleep account in advance of known sleep disruptions (such as going on a long trip) or when we know that we are entering a period of sleep disruption or heightened stress. I do this when I am anticipating international travel.

• Now to the key finding of the commission: We have up to seven days (or nights) to make up any sleep overdraft we might have accumulated in the previous week. If we don't make it up, the overdraft penalty cannot be redeemed. This means that catching that extra sleep on a Saturday or Sunday afternoon may be a lot healthier for us than we realize! It's probably the last opportunity you have to make up for sleep lost during the past week.

The bottom-line message from the sleep commission's report is simply this: Most of us can improve our physical and emotional health dramatically, if we just try to balance our sleep bank account on a weekly basis.

Sleep Deficit May Become Permanent

Let me draw your attention to another consequence of insufficient sleep. Recently, sleep research has opened yet a more alarming door. It has been discovered that both humans and animals who have chronic sleep deprivation can reach a point at which their ability to catch up on lost sleep is lost forever. This means that the consequences of sleep deprivation can be permanent.[4] I don't know about you, but it is a frightening prospect to contemplate this sort of consequence for our families.

Over time, nights of missed sleep, whether caused by a sleep disorder or simply not scheduling enough time for the necessary zzz's, can build into a severe sleep deficit that cannot be made up. Sleep experts call this a "sleep debt."

While it is extremely difficult to measure someone's sleep debt, there is one home strategy you can use with your child or teenager, or for yourself for that matter. During the daytime, find a quiet place where you, or your child, can relax for a while. No phones or music players, just sit by yourself and relax. Now wait and see what happens. If the feeling of sleep comes fairly easily and quickly, you probably have some sleep debt. One should be able to sit still for a while during the day, say for at least five minutes without any stimulation, and not feel sleepy.

Now let me outline some strategies for managing your sleep account.

Managing Your Sleep Account

You need to take managing your sleep account as seriously as you take managing your money account. Neglecting either can be disastrous. Just as paying attention to every penny you spend keeps you solvent, so paying attention to every minute you sleep can keep you healthy.

With millions of dollars each year going toward advertising the latest sleep aid or pill, it's not surprising that many have lost sight of the importance of simple behavioral changes that can make a world of difference to their sleep habits. Not every sleep problem we struggle with needs a pill. While medication can be helpful and give your sleep problems a quick, though temporary, fix, there are other effective psychotherapies that are longer lasting and free of side effects and addiction. One approach, called cognitive/behavioral therapy (CBT), is widely used here. It is this CBT approach that I will tie into your sleep account management here.

Basics of Sleep-Bank Management

Losing one hour of sleep a day accumulates to a loss of seven hours over a week—the equivalent of a whole night's sleep debt. Or, putting it the other way, if you sleep one hour longer every night, you add almost a whole night's sleep a week. To help you overcome your sleep debt, I will describe four strategies:

1. Increasing your total sleep time
2. Preventing sleep overdrafts
3. Preventing "sleep thefts"
4. Building up "sleep equity"

Increasing Your Total Sleep Time

I'm not so naive as to think that you can go from sleeping only six or seven hours a night to, say eight and a half or nine hours a night, with just the snap of a finger. Our sleeping habits become deeply programmed into our brains, and it will take some time to modify them. So be patient as you persevere. It took me at least two years to go from sleeping about six hours a night to what is now my regular sleep schedule of nine hours. At times I thought I would never make it. Now I cannot function without my full nine hours of sleep.

Confirmation of my new sleep pattern came about five years ago when I had to have bypass surgery. I come from a family burdened with heart disease—as mentioned earlier. My father died of heart disease, as did an uncle. I have a brother who has had several heart attacks and bypass surgeries. So it was a great relief for me to discover through a routine screening exam, and without having had a heart attack, that I needed surgery to repair some blockages. My surgery went well, and my surgeon and I struck up a relationship afterward. He would come chat with me in the hospital between his other surgeries.

During one of our chats he shared with me that something had changed in my heart arteries about 25 or 30 years ago. It looked as if I had stopped building up soft plaque (the gunk that blocks the arteries). The plaque in my arteries had mainly calcified, which is why a CT scan discovered it during a regular checkup. So he wanted to know what changed all those years ago, and possibly saved my life. I reflected for a moment, and then realized that it was about that time that I started regularly sleeping nine hours a night. While there are no studies that show this, and I may be wrong, I am convinced that this change made the difference in my life.

Earlier in the book, I described a way in which you can determine how much sleep you need by adding small amounts of sleep and observing how it affects your performance and feeling of well-being. I will follow the same "incremental" model here as I describe a way for permanently lengthening your sleep duration, even if you did not do the test I described. If you know you have a problem and want to sleep longer, here is how you should proceed:

First decide how much extra sleep time you want to add and settle on a goal for your new sleep pattern. Let's say you sleep six and a half hours a night now. You set your first goal at eight hours. Later, once you have achieved success here, you might try for more.

The added sleep time is one and a half hours. This is, not surprisingly, quite a big leap, so we need to break it down into smaller increments. The key to success in changing all habits is to take it one small step at a time—a baby step! It's easier to master and become habituated to a small change than a big one. Big steps usually breed backsliders—as everyone who struggles to lose weight knows!

Now you must decide whether you add the extra time to the start or the end of your allotted sleep time. If you are already getting up just in time to go to work, then it must be at the start end. So for the next two weeks, consistently go to bed 15 minutes earlier every night. Perhaps you can convince the family to do the same—especially your teenagers. This might take some creative incentives, but it's worth it.

As mentioned earlier, you should begin with about 15 minutes. Once you are sleeping an extra 15 minutes regularly (for more than two weeks), then add another 15 minutes. Don't be too impulsive here or you will end up backsliding! When your goal is completed, you will have made six manageable baby steps and have built a new sleep pattern.

Preventing Sleep Overdrafts

The next step toward building a healthier sleep account is to pay attention to little losses of sleep as soon as they occur. When I was a child my mother would often say, "Watch the pennies, and the pounds will take care of themselves." Or the American equivalent would be, "Pay attention to the cents, and the dollars will take care of themselves!" Regarding sleep accounts, I suppose one could say, "Pay attention to the minutes you sleep, and the hours slept will take care of themselves."

You prevent a sleep overdraft by avoiding the little losses in sleep, and then making up for any time lost as soon as possible. In essence, don't let your sleep debt accumulate. If you couldn't sleep last night, record how much sleep you lost, then add one-third of the lost sleep time to each of the next three nights. For example, let's say that for whatever reason (barking dogs, teenage kids coming home late, or just some worry on your mind), you estimate that you lost about one and a half hours of your normal sleep last night. Well, one and a half hours divided by three is half an hour. So, for the next three nights, add half an hour to your sleep time.

Spreading this out over three nights means you are not making too radical a change. And even if all you do is just lie and relax, you are building a habit that will stand you in good stead the rest of your life. I do this all the time!

But let's say that you lost sleep several nights in a row. This happens when you have a sick child or have to drive through the night to get somewhere urgently. This is more complicated. You must figure out how much extra sleep you can reasonably allot yourself for each of the next seven nights, and then add the extra sleep time to each of these nights to make up for the loss. Remember that the key period for making up a sleep loss is seven days—but fortunately this always includes a weekend.

If you haven't been able to sleep a full night for a long time now, your situation is obviously more serious. Just adding a half hour or hour to your nightly sleep isn't going to repair the damage. Your overdraft is too large, so you may have to just declare sleep bankruptcy and start a new sleep account cycle. To do this requires a more serious strategy and even, possibly, changing your lifestyle to overcome not just your tendency to create a sleep debt but your sleep disorder as well.

Preventing "Sleep Thefts"

All banks are vulnerable to thieves, and your sleep account is no exception. Just as robbers can steal your money, there are sleep robbers that can deplete your sleep bank.

Family Sleep Robbers

What are the leading sleep-deprivation culprits, besides late-night TV and the Internet? Experts routinely point their finger at needy kids and snoring spouses. About one-half of all parents have their sleep disturbed an average of twice a week because their child wakens them during the night. In a baby's first year of life a parent can lose up to two hundred hours of sleep! The good news is that there are solutions for these top two shut-eye robbers.

How can you balance the late-night mommy or daddy beat with your slumber needs? First, couples need to learn how to take shifts so that it is not always the mother who has to struggle. It's possible Mom is breastfeeding and therefore has to wake up. But for those cases where parents are bottle feeding, partners need to take turns so that one is not always responsible for tending to children in the middle of the night. Some sleep-deprived mothers pump and save breast milk ahead of time so that Dad can help feed when she's too exhausted.

If you're a so-called morning person, take the 3 AM shift onward, and go to bed a bit earlier (say 9 to 10 PM if possible). Your nighttime partner can take the 9 PM to midnight shift. Hopefully, everyone will be asleep from midnight to 3 AM—babies included! If your sleep is consistently disrupted because you have to put an older child back to bed several times each night, then it's okay to consider letting him or her into your bed—but for a limited time only. I know that this is a bit contentious, but reality must sometimes prevail. As long as you don't make a habit of it, when a child is sick it can be comforting for him or her to stay with you for a short time, and then be encouraged to go back to bed. Make it a habit to reward your kids for staying in their beds most of the time.

The Snoring Spouse Robber

Snoring forces many partners to sleep in another room—and it can be a major cause of conflict. Whether your partner snores loudly, tosses and turns, or simply has a different shut-eye schedule, dealing with a bad bed partner can be a challenge. There is absolutely no reason why you should let a snoring spouse rob you of sleep. To improve your sleep (and possibly help save your marriage), keep a few "buffers" on hand, such as eye covers and earplugs. These will help dim any light or drown out any noise caused by your partner. If your spouse has a serious snoring problem, encourage him or her to have a sleep evaluation to rule out sleep apnea.

On the topic of snoring, a popular remedy now being touted is the use of "nasal strips." Applied to the outside of the nose, they are supposed to open your nasal passages. However, there is much dispute over whether they really do this. Furthermore, most snoring occurs at the back of the throat, so opening nasal passages may help improve breathing, say if you have a cold and you are congested, but whether or not they can cure snoring is another matter. They are often used by athletes in order to increase oxygen intake, and depending on your nose's design, they may just help. If you are a snorer, you may want to try them to see if they work for you. I will wait until I see some more definitive research on the matter.

The Temperature Robber

Conflicts over the sleep environment can also be a sleep robber. You like it hot, but your partner likes it cool. The ideal bedroom sleeping temperature is between 68 and 74 degrees, if this will settle any arguments, so try and split the difference. My wife and I prefer 78 degrees in summer and winter. But this is California! Consider an electric blanket for only one side of the bed, or a thick quilt on one side and a thin one on the other.

The Caffeine Robber

I've already discussed caffeine's demons, so I list it here only for completeness. Many people unintentionally create a vicious caffeine merry-go-round. They can't get to sleep at night because they've had too much caffeine, and then because they are so exhausted the next day, they have to reach for their caffeine fix to keep them going. And they repeat the cycle over and over again. If you are going to stay out of sleep debt, you have to get off this merry-go-round.

The "Lack of Exercise" Robber

Good sleep requires a tired body, not just a fatigued mind. Do you get enough exercise during the day? Some people have a hard time sleeping or staying asleep because their bodies are not getting enough physical exertion to fatigue them. They spend long hours sitting at computers or behind desks, then go home to sit some more in front of the TV. Our modern life is completely out of touch with the fact that our bodies were made to move. Our brains have outsmarted us and found ways for us to sit and work. If this is your life, get up and move! A lot!

If you don't get some physical exercise each day, your sleep bank is being robbed. Even just taking an evening stroll around a few blocks can be a great sleep inducer. However, more vigorous exercise is important for keeping our hearts and lungs in good shape. If you exercise at night, make sure to leave adequate recovery time before going to bed to allow your body to unwind. This will help you make a bigger and better deposit in your sleep bank.

Building Up "Sleep Equity"

The amount of sleep needed for a particular individual is dependent on not only that person's age but also his or her biological makeup. Sleep debt has been likened to writing a check for an amount greater than what you have available in your bank account. But you can counter a bank overdraft by building up sleep equity—adding more sleep ahead.

If your life is such that you can never be certain just how much sleep you can expect, or that it is not possible for you to regularly sleep the same amount of hours every night, then what you need to do is set aside more sleep time when you can. In other words, build up a healthy sleep reserve at every opportunity. Then if your sleep is disrupted for whatever reason, it's not going to affect you much, as you would have prepaid your sleep debt. In other words, you can use the "seven-day rule" for making up lost sleep and apply it proactively—that is, by building up your sleep equity ahead of time. It's like putting a larger cash balance in your checking account just in case unexpected sleep expenses come along.

I do this when I have to travel internationally. I know ahead of time that my sleep schedule will be changed the moment I step on the plane. So without fail, when preparing for a trip, I intentionally sleep one extra hour (sometimes it is one and a half hours) every night for the week preceding my trip. With my sleep equity fully stocked, I can weather the sleep time lost without difficulty. What a difference it can make to tiresome travel!

Then there are those who serve us in some special way and who need to maintain alertness and performance under challenging circumstances—such as police, firefighters, rescue workers, armed services personnel, physicians, and so on. They often suffer from severe sleep disruptions with serious consequences. They, too, can maintain or improve their performance by building up sleep equity. This may mean having to sleep in multiple short bouts throughout the day, but if they follow the basic sleep rules for making up sleep over a seven-day period or depositing sleep ahead of time, they should be able to keep their sleep balance in the black.

Newborn Babies and Your Sleep Bank

Of all the challenges facing young couples, none is more challenging from a sleep perspective than having a new baby in the family. Managing your sleep bank as a couple can be particularly difficult at this time. Whether it is your first or your fourth child, this glorious and memorable time of your life demands adjustment and will test your endurance as much as, or perhaps more than, any other life challenge.

My purpose here is not to provide a comprehensive plan for newborn childcare; I'll leave that to the baby experts. I merely want to offer a few sleep-related principles that can help you manage your sleep bank when you have the glorious gift of a newborn on the scene.

- Tailor your own sleep plan to fit the needs of your baby. Listen to and watch your baby carefully. You have to learn to distinguish "awake" crying (baby is ventilating his or her lungs) from "hunger" crying (baby is demanding food). This is where my wife and I struggled with our first baby. My wife was determined to breastfeed her. But she seemed to cry all the time, and we couldn't tell the difference between "awake" and "hunger" crying. After several weeks of total sleep loss by both of us, I decided to weigh our baby before and after each feeding. We discovered that she wasn't getting enough milk. A quick consultation with our doctor confirmed that we needed to supplement her milk—and peace descended from heaven. We could actually get four hours of blissful sleep at a time.

- Help your baby distinguish night from day. A newborn needs 16 to 18 hours sleep a day. At first it is evenly distributed, but as the baby grows it helps to have him or her sleep in a well-lit room during the day and a dark room at night. Some parents make the mistake of having their baby sleep in a darkened room during the day. By letting your baby sleep in daylight, he or she will gradually develop nocturnal variation sensitivity.

- As your baby grows older, learn the signs of tiredness and put the baby down to sleep when she's ready for it. Otherwise she will be very unhappy. Signs include quieting down, losing interest in toys, ignoring people nearby, and causing a fuss. Our babies would throw their toys out of the crib when they were ready to sleep.

  Also, teach infants the art of falling asleep on their own. Put them to bed when they are drowsy but not fully asleep. This creates a better sleep hygiene than putting them to bed when they are already asleep.

- If you have other children, protect them from possible sleep disruptions. You can do this by improving sound insulation, such as putting a towel along the bottom of doors, or even having older children sleep with earplugs.

- Mom, if you're breastfeeding, make yourself as comfortable as possible for the nighttime feed. Even if you're awake, try to rest your body. And as I mentioned, if you aren't breastfeeding, have your spouse take turns bottle feeding, allowing yourself periodic respite.

Tips for Getting Back to Sleep

Whether you're a mom who's juggling a career with raising a family, or a dad with a challenging job, or a couple with a newborn, we all, myself included, suffer periodic wakings in the early hours of the morning, and then struggle to get back to sleep again. Here are some tips that can help you get back to sleep when awakened:

- First, master a few of the relaxation exercises, such as can be found on my Relaxation CD described in Appendix D, and practice them while lying there, waiting to go back to sleep. Relaxation is the best way to lower your adrenaline and make you sleepy.
- Try visualization and imagination exercises (also on the CD). One effective way to distract an overactive mind is to visualize and imagine things. For instance, rearrange yourself in bed so you are lying comfortably on your back. Now focus all your attention on your toes and visualize walking down an endless stairwell. Keep your eyes on your feet. Thinking about repetitive or mindless activities like this will distract your brain and help it to shut down and adjust to sleep. It's not unlike the proverbial "counting sheep" strategy—which, by the way, can also work.
- Consider changing your bedtime. If you are experiencing sleeplessness or insomnia consistently, think about going to bed at a different time. If you are going to bed late, try going to bed earlier. Your anxiety about not getting enough sleep may be keeping you awake.

Ten Ways to Improve the Quality of Your Sleep

No matter your age or what your sleep problem is, here are ten suggestions for improving the quality of your sleep. Copy this list and pin it up where all members of your family can see it. The principles underlying each of these suggestions are explained in different sections of this book.

1. Go to bed at the same time every night.
2. Keep your bedroom as dark, quiet, and comfortable as possible.
3. Drink no caffeine-based drink after 3 PM (preferably eliminate all caffeine).
4. Learn a relaxation technique (offered at the end of this book) and use it when going to sleep.
5. About an hour before bedtime, turn down all lights and darken your environment.
6. Do not engage in any exciting activity after 8 PM (stay away from your computer). (However, sex is still fine.)
7. Get up every morning at the same time (after having had enough sleep) and get into sunlight as soon as possible.
8. If you wake up at night, try not to get up. If you must, get back into bed as soon as possible and don't turn on any bright light.
9. Make sure you exercise or do enough physical work every day to make you tired.
10. Work hard at stress management and de-stress yourself before going to bed. High stress is our greatest sleep killer.

Go Easy on Sleeping Pills

Sleep that knits up the ravelled sleave of care
The death of each day's life, sore labour's bath
Balm of hurt minds, great nature's second course,
Chief nourisher in life's feast.
—WILLIAM SHAKESPEARE, *MACBETH*

According to the advertisements you see on television, the best solution to a sleep problem lies in a sleeping pill. The ads make the "pill solution" look so simple, tantalizing, effective, and innocent. Not surprisingly, therefore, manufacturing sleeping pills is big business—whether it's a real sleeping pill or nothing more than a placebo! Regrettably, consumers may rely too much on sleeping pills and overlook safer, non-drug, and cheaper remedies, according to an article from *Consumer Reports*.[1]

How common is it to use sleeping pills? About 43 million prescriptions for sleeping pills were filled in the United States during 2005, up 32 percent from 2001, according to the *Consumer Reports'* "Best Buy Drugs" report.[2] By now it's probably a lot higher. And many more take nonprescription sleep aids as well.

Sleeping pills are both a blessing and a curse. They are a blessing, for instance, when you are experiencing a bad circumstance in your life, if you are in pain, or when there are unavoidable interruptions and you need to get sleep at any cost. I have several patients who right now could not survive without the help of a sleep medication. It is what keeps them sane. Whether you have been let go from your job, are worried about your future, have experienced a recent bereavement, or are facing major surgery, a sedative can help you through these troubling times. No harm is done by using an artificial sedative here, provided it is only taken for a short period of time—say a week or two.

But many people who consume sleeping pills today are not in a major life crisis. They are over-stressed or have another chronic cause of sleeplessness. And this is a different story. Sleeping pills are not the long-term answer here, and can even become a curse when used indiscriminately and without limits. They may disguise the problem, but they do not solve it. Still worse, they can create a new problem: dependence. I have seen patients who, despite their sincerest efforts, could no longer sleep without an aid after just a few weeks of continuous use of sleeping pills.

Patients vary, of course, in how quickly they become dependent on a sleeping pill. Most artificial sleep inducers take over and displace the brain's natural sleep messengers, and it doesn't take long before you become totally dependent on them. And if you then try to stop using the artificial sleep aid, the starved brain rebels and one cannot fall asleep naturally again. It's called "rebound insomnia."

So, while there are times when it is appropriate to use a sleeping pill, if you persist in taking them, it is only a matter of time before you become dependent, even addicted. How does such an addiction come about when all doctors know that artificial sleep aids can become addicting and that, except in rare cases, a patient should only take them for a short period? Some patients play games with their physicians. Some years ago, a patient of mine educated me in how she was able to get around the obstacles. She set up four different doctors, each believing that he or she was the only physician she was seeing, to prescribe a round of sleeping pills.

When the first doctor became resistant to prescribing any more sleeping pills for her, she moved on to the next—and the next. Then when she was finished with the fourth doctor, she started back with the first, who believed, of course, that she had not been taking sleeping pills since he last consulted with her a year before. This way she could rotate through the doctors with a continuous supply of powerful sedatives, and none of them suspected she was abusing the drugs. She also used four different pharmacies, carefully avoiding more than one in a chain where all records are centralized. She didn't consult me originally for her addiction problem and it only came to light unintentionally. It took two years of psychotherapy to break her addiction.

But I also have some good news here. I have seen many patients who, with just a little effort, have broken their dependence on sleeping pills before they became seriously addicted, and now rejoice in their newfound freedom. So even if you are dependent on a sleep aid, it need not become a permanent dependence. You can certainly avoid it becoming an addiction, as we will see. However, if you are already addicted to sleeping pills, I urge you to see an addictions specialist right away.

Sleeping Pill Confusion

It is easy to be confused about sedatives, sleeping pills, and sleep aids. They are all sedatives, but sleeping pills are more powerful and usually prescribed, while sleep aids are nonprescription. Sleeping pills are being touted every day in TV ads, so many become accustomed to the idea that if you have a sleep problem, all you have to do is ask your doctor for a sleeping pill. Because over-the-counter sleep aids don't require a doctor's prescription, many people turn to them on a regular basis, and at the slightest prospect of a bad night.

Within moderation this is not a problem. When you have had an unusually demanding day and your mind is racing like mad, a sleep aid can be a great blessing. Or if you're going through a temporary life crisis and need your sleep to be able to function, a short-term prescription sleep aid might be quite appropriate. So please don't take what I am saying here as a total ban on all sleep aids. Far from it, as I would be condemning myself. International travel is particularly sleep challenging for me, and a sleep aid has often been a lifesaver.

There are also a host of "natural" and health food supplements that are hyped as the ultimate solution to every sleep problem you can imagine. And finally, there is my grandmother's remedy: "Archie, do lots of exercise and have a clear conscience, and you will never suffer from insomnia," as she pushed me out the door to go and play. As a boy I didn't always sleep peacefully. But today I know what she meant and sleep better because of her advice.

Before looking at specific sleep aids and evaluating them, here are a few basic principles to keep in mind when using sleeping pills:

- No sleeping pill yet invented can cure insomnia. They only provide palliative and temporary relief.
- Major prescription sleep medications should never be taken without a careful evaluation by your doctor. Where possible, try an over-the-counter sleep aid first, but be aware that these also have some risks.
- Don't believe everything you read in advertisements, hear on the radio, or see on TV. A lot of it is sales hype, and sometimes gives a false sense of security and confidence in taking sleep aids.
- Sleep medications are only moderately helpful in the short run and lose their effectiveness with long-term use.
- Insomnia invariably returns when the medications are discontinued, oftentimes worse than before. For this reason, you should never stop sleeping pills suddenly.

• If you suffer from a mild, occasional insomnia, first try a non-drug treatment. Several behavioral therapies are available that teach ways to improve sleep habits. Also, the relaxation exercises described in Appendix D provide a healthier road to better sleep.

• Sleepwalking, sleep-driving, and even sleep-eating may occur when someone is taking a prescription sedative.

Go Easy on Sedating Pills

Because they are so common, you need to know the pros, cons, and risks associated with sedating medications (both prescription and non-prescription), before you start to take them. You also need to know whether your particular sleep problem is suited to such treatment.

What hazards are linked to sedatives?

• Long term, they reduce your ability to return to natural sleep. For short-term insomnia it is better to try to sleep without medication, even if it means enduring a few nights of sleeplessness.

• While sleep drugs help us sleep and are not necessarily harmful to healthy adults, they make the brain's sleep mechanism "lazy." One never feels refreshed after a night of artificial sleep.

• Depending on the type of sleep medication used, different parts of normal sleep architecture will be disturbed. Some medications reduce dreaming, and therefore disturb your brain's ability to reorganize itself. Others increase dream sleep at the expense of your non-dream sleep. This imbalance leaves you feeling unrested when you wake up. Often, I wake up with a headache when my sleep isn't balanced.

• Like all drugs, sleeping pills have multiple side effects, and these can outweigh their benefits.

Types of Sedatives

There are a number of different sedatives on the market now, and new aids are arriving all the time. I sure hope that one day we will have the perfect sleeping pill that is safe, non-addicting, and gives us the complete sleep nature intends us to have. But we are a long way from such an Eden. This means that it's imperative for parents to know something about the sedatives available today, especially before letting their kids take them.

Figure 7 on the next page summarizes the major sleep aids available today—prescription, nonprescription, naturals, and herbals. The table indicates how each aid works, what it offers, and the pros and cons of taking it.

It's quite a long list, so let me provide a brief descriptive overview so you can make informed decisions about which to use and which to avoid.

There are basically six types of sedating medications. Each has advantages and disadvantages. Some are used for serious sleep disorders, some for minor sleep disruptions. I am not including a group of drugs called "hypnotics" (such as barbiturates or opiates). They are anesthetics. But anesthesia is not natural sleep. They are also very habit forming, seldom used outside a hospital, and not suited to treating everyday insomnia or common sleep problems. So I consider them to be outside the scope of this book.

Nonprescription Sleep Aids

These are available over the counter and usually contain an antihistamine that makes you drowsy and helps you fall asleep. While they are quite effective for mild insomnia, you should keep in mind that any antihistamine must be used with caution.

What are antihistamines? Well, as the name implies they are "anti" histamines. Histamines are substances that try to attach themselves to

KNOW YOUR SLEEP MEDICATIONS

1. Nonprescription Sleep Aids

Names	How They Work	Pros	Cons
Benadryl Nytol Tylenol PM Sominex Sleep-Eze Nyquil	Contains antihistamine that makes you drowsy.	Over-the-counter	Short-term use only; Morning grogginess; Reduces dream sleep; Dry mouth; Dizziness

2. Prescription Sleep Aids—BENZODIAZEPINES (Tranquilizers)

Names	How They Work	Pros	Cons
Restoril Dalmane Halcion Doral	Enhances brain's tranquilizers, reducing alertness, causing sedation and muscle relaxation.	Induces sleep. Reduces anxiety.	Addicting in long term; Morning hangover; Rebound insomnia; Many side effects

3. Prescription Sleep Aids—NON-BENZODIAZEPINES

Names	How They Work	Pros	Cons
Ambien Ambien CR Sonata Lunesta	Increases GABA, which is sleep inducing.	More effective. Short acting. Safer and less side effects.	Addicting in long term; Side effects like drowsiness, dizziness, and headaches

4. Prescription Sleep Aids—MELATONIN RECEPTOR AGONISTS

Names	How They Work	Pros	Cons
Rozerem	Acts on brain's melatonin receptor to induce sleep.	Non-narcotic. Fffective for sleep onset problems.	Exacerbates depression; Dizziness, upset stomach, change in food taste

5. Prescription Sleep Aids—SEDATING ANTIDEPRESSANTS

Names	How They Work	Pros	Cons
Elavil Endep Sinequan Desyrel	Several antidepressants have sedating side effects and can be used for sleep.	Non-narcotic. Effective for sleep onset problems.	Side effects: dry mouth, dizziness, upset stomach, weight gain, sexual dysfunction

6. "Natural" and Herbal Sleep Aids:

Names	How They Work	Pros	Cons
Melatonin Valerian Kava kava	Animal or synthetic Herbal	Nonprescription	Quality not controlled

FIGURE 7: Know Your Sleep Medications

the cells in your body—and then irritate them. Every person who suffers from allergies knows them well; they are the source of their allergy discomfort. Histamines can cause itching, sneezing, a runny nose, and watery eyes—typical symptoms of an allergic reaction. So antihistamines, therefore, prevent these allergic histamines from attaching to your cells, and only as a bonus can make you drowsy as well—a boon for mild and occasional insomniacs.

But remember, when you aren't suffering from allergies and you are using them only for sleep, you are essentially using the side effect of the drug, not its main function. In other words, it will do more than just help you fall asleep. So always keep this in mind and limit your use of them. For instance, while antihistamines aren't a serious threat for healthy adults, they can be a problem for older adults, young children, or anyone with a health problem. Also, remember that they can affect your ability to drive or operate machines. (Read the small print on the label.) They can befuddle your thinking and cause your mouth and eyes to feel dry—so only take them at bedtime. Do not "double dose," as it will prolong the drug's sedating effect into the next day. Also, avoid alcohol when taking them, as it can increase your drowsiness. However, for some people, antihistamines have the opposite effect and can cause nervousness, restlessness, or insomnia.

Prescription Sleeping Pills—Benzodiazepine Based

These are the most commonly prescribed sleep aids. Hypnotic benzodiazepines (they are, in effect, tranquilizers) have strong sedative effects and are often prescribed for the short-term management of insomnia. They do not reduce your dream sleep—and this is important. However, they differ in the amount of time they stay active in your body. Some have a quick onset; others are slow. Your doctor will decide which of them suits your needs. Longer-acting benzodiazepines have side effects, including drowsiness, that may persist well into the next day, whereas intermediate-acting benzodiazepines may have less of a "hang-over" effect.

Older people cannot metabolize (break down and remove) these drugs very well, so they may experience prolonged drowsiness the next day, with an increased risk of falling or accidents. So the elderly should only take short-acting benzodiazepines. Of course, even a short-acting benzodiazepine will increase the risk of falling while it is working. Is it better to spend a sleepless night in your own bed, or a sleepless night in the emergency room with a broken hip? You may not agree with this dogmatic approach, but it is what a doctor should ask an elderly patient who wants a sleeping pill.

The important point to remember here is this: Pay careful attention to how you feel the next day. If your "hangover" is drowsy, either the drug is lasting too long or you took it too late. Go to bed earlier, or request a shorter-acting drug. Remember, each of us has a unique reaction to all drugs. Some drugs hang around much longer in some of us than in others.

Also remember, benzodiazepine-based hypnotics are usually reserved for short-term treatment of acute sleep problems only. They are not a substitute for psychotherapy and stress management, or other behavioral strategies that can help you deal with the anxiety that might be keeping you awake at night. Tolerance (when a drug loses its power) and dependence (when you cannot do without a drug) will occur if these benzodiazepines are taken regularly for more than just a few weeks, so be cautious and set limits.

Prescription Sleeping Pills—Non-Benzodiazepine Based

Here we have some of the newer sleep medications that are not tranquilizers in the usual sense. They are better for serious or prolonged sleep problems. But this does not mean that they are any less of a problem themselves. For instance, some people just cannot tolerate them. They experience bizarre side effects. Some report that they work well; in others, they do not. It is somewhat of a mixed bag right now.

On the positive side, this group of sleep medications is generally associated with a lower risk of abuse than the benzodiazepines. Although these medications are safer than the benzodiazepines, they should not be used on a long-term basis. Lunesta is an exception, as it is approved for longer-term use. However, since it is quite new, we have yet to see whether users become so dependent on it that they have to take the drug forever.

You should also keep in mind that these medications will not address your family member's underlying problems—physical or mental—that might be the cause of their insomnia. For instance, on the physical side, sleep-related breathing disorders (sleep apnea), restless legs syndrome (RLS), and chronic pain are not fixed. And on the emotional side, severe depression or anxiety will remain unaffected.

Prescription Sleeping Pills: Melatonin Receptor Based

Rozerem (ramelteon) is a prescription insomnia medication that was approved by the FDA in July 2005, and began to be marketed to consumers in 2006. Rozerem has a unique mechanism of action. It is called a "melatonin receptor agonist," which simply means that it works by attaching to melatonin receptors in your brain. It selectively targets specific receptors in the brain that are responsible for controlling the body's sleep/wake cycle and works by mimicking your brain's natural melatonin. (You can find more information about Rozerem at: http://www .rozerem.com/en/about_rozerem/prescribing_information/.)

Rozerem may have an advantage over the other sleep medications for the following reasons:

- It specifically targets the brain structures responsible for the sleep/wake cycle.

- It is the first and only prescription sleep medication that has shown no evidence of abuse, dependence, or withdrawal (and, therefore, it has not been designated as a controlled substance by the U.S. Drug Enforcement Agency).
- Rozerem is approved by the FDA for long-term use in adults (but not children as of yet).

But there are no drugs without a downside. Some of the primary warnings and contraindications for Rozerem include the following:

- It is not recommended for use in anyone with severe sleep apnea.
- It should not be used in patients with severe liver problems or sensitivity to the medication.
- It must not be taken with alcohol.
- The more common side effects include daytime carry-over sleepiness, dizziness, and fatigue.
- There may be a worsening of depression, including suicidal ideation. Also, hallucinations and nightmares may occur.

Prescription Sleep Aids—Sedating Antidepressants

Here is another form of sleep medication that is widely used. Insomnia is quite common in depression. When antidepressants first came out, it was found that some of them not only relieved the depression but helped patients to sleep better as well. I have recommended this approach often to patients. Sedating antidepressants are used in lower doses than in depression—so make sure you draw your doctor's attention to this should you want to try this approach. The sedating antidepressants most commonly used to help with sleep include Trazodone (Desyrel), Amitriptyline (Elavil), and Doxepin (Sinequan). But please remember that some of the side effects of these medications can be problematic for the elderly. For instance, they can cause a heart block or orthostatic hypotension (get dizzy when you stand up) in some patients, especially those who are elderly or have cardiovascular disease, so please discuss these issues carefully with your doctor. If your doctor determines that it is safe for you to take these medications, there are benefits of using them for sleep:

- They are non-addicting.
- They do not produce physical dependence or tolerance.
- They have the added benefit of providing some analgesic effect (pain-relieving properties).
- They generally have a low incidence of side effects, especially when used in low doses.

Some individuals do experience adverse side effects, including dry mouth, blurred vision, a "hangover" in the morning, constipation, urinary retention, and/or nausea, but these effects can be reduced by lowering the dosage after a short time.

"Natural" and Herbal Sleep Aids

These are the more contentious sleep aids, because there are no regulatory controls over their use, nor is their manufacturing monitored for safety. You need to make sure you are buying them from a reputable supplier. Many sleep sufferers have found relief from "natural" and "herbal" remedies. So, if they work for you, why not use them? Research on their effectiveness is still under way, so the jury is still out on whether they really do aid sleep or whether they offer just a sleep placebo. Since they are not cheap, we really do need controlled studies to determine their efficacy. More importantly, the safety of these products, and the extent to which they interact with other medications, has not been established and little is really known about them. Nonetheless, many choose to use them.

One natural sleep aid that is receiving a lot of attention lately is called melatonin. Melatonin, as you will recall, is what the pineal gland in the brain puts out when darkness arrives. It helps us sleep. It's the same hormone that makes animals hibernate in winter.

The FDA classifies melatonin as a food supplement, so there is no regulatory control. While many use it for insomnia, the FDA has only approved it for "delayed sleep phase disorder"—a fancy name for jetlag! In plain language, it is only recommended to help you get over time changes while traveling. I have used it several times for this purpose, and it seems to work quite effectively, if you take it shortly before bedtime in your new time zone—at least, it's effective for the first few days. Thereafter, there is little scientific evidence that melatonin has a role in promoting healthy sleep habits or treating any form of sleep disorder.

Melatonin supplements (in pill form) are now readily available as over-the-counter aids. However, there are two types of melatonin: natural (taken from the pineal gland of animals) and synthetic (man-made). Since it is possible for animal melatonin to be contaminated with a virus, many experts don't recommend it. The synthetic form of melatonin does not pose this risk, though it may not be as effective. If you are not sure what form of melatonin you have, whether it's natural or synthetic, ask your pharmacist. Also, several new natural sleep aids, combining melatonin with other herbals, are now starting to appear. I have no idea how effective they are.

Just like every substance you put in your mouth, melatonin also has side effects. Among those reported are excessive sleepiness, headaches, a "heavy-head" feeling, stomach discomfort, depression, and feeling "hung over" the next day. Further study is needed to find out more about melatonin's side effects, especially those that are delayed or have long-term damaging effects.

Breaking the Sleeping Pill Habit

While it is important that you know as much as possible about the sleep aids you and/or your family are using, it is equally important to know when to stop and how to break your dependence on sleep aids—

natural, prescription, or nonprescription. I have encountered dozens of people who, after finding relief for their sleep problem, discovered that they have gone from the frying pan into the fire. The pill that once helped them get to sleep now makes it impossible for them to sleep without it. They have become entrapped by a pill that now rules their lives. Amazing how much power a little pill like this can have over you!

Taking a sleep aid on a regular basis, prescription or nonprescription, shuts down the brain's naturally produced sedatives, and this modifies your brain's sleep onset mechanism. In a sense, your brain becomes lazy and relies entirely on the added help it gets from the sedatives. Then if you stop the artificial sleep aid, there is nothing to take its place. It takes several days, even weeks, after stopping the aid before the brain's factories come back on line and provide its natural sedative. And it's for this reason that breaking your dependence on a sleep aid should be gradual, as we will see.

Before proceeding, however, I need to emphasize that if you want to stop a prescription sleeping aid that you've been taking on a regular basis, it is essential that you discuss your intention with your physician before you start. Stopping some sedatives suddenly can be hazardous. It not only causes rebound insomnia, but more seriously, puts you at increased risk for seizures. So make sure you seek your physician's approval to proceed, and consider any guidance your doctor may offer. My strategies here should only be followed with your physician's approval, and modified with whatever suggestions your physician offers.

In addition to securing your physician's advice, you may find it beneficial to seek some counseling help as well. Sleep medications can create a powerful psychological dependence, in addition to the physical. The most effective therapeutic approach here is cognitive behavioral therapy (CBT). One study using this approach found that 85 percent of long-term users of sedative hypnotic drugs were able to free themselves.[3] This is very good news. It is this approach I will describe in the exercises to follow.

There are three important principles to keep in mind as you try to reduce your dependence on sleep aids:

1. You must taper off your sleep aids very slowly and at a rate with which you feel comfortable. Reducing a sleep aid can produce some anxiety, and this anxiety can intensify your difficulty falling sleep.

2. Prepare yourself for some setbacks. While some can waltz through their tapering without a misstep, others will have periodic setbacks. If you find that your tapering fails at some point, go back to the last successful step in the process and stay there for a few nights until all is stabilized; then proceed from there.

3. Be prepared to encounter some withdrawal reactions. Becoming dependent on a sleep aid is not unlike an addiction. Your brain will miss the sleep aid each time you lower it and will kick up a fuss for a while. So be patient and try to ignore the withdrawal symptoms if they are minor. If they are bothersome, don't move to the next step for a few days, and seek counsel if necessary.

Here are the basic steps you need to follow:

1. For the first week, keep a careful record of exactly how often you use a sleep aid and how many pills you take. This will provide you with a "baseline" so you will know where you are beginning.

2. For the second week, choose a night when it will be convenient for you to lower the sleep aid dose. Choose a night that doesn't require any special action the following day. For example, don't choose a night before an important business meeting or a day you will be traveling— you will need all the sleep you can get! Preferably, it should be over a weekend or before you have a day off—say a Friday night.

3. For the selected night, cut your dose of the sleep aid in half, and only take this amount. If you normally take two pills, then take only one. If you take one pill, then take half a pill. Do this only for this selected night. Take your normal dose for the rest of the week. For every night of the week, whether you are taking your normal dose or the modified dose, make it a habit to do a relaxation exercise (see Relaxation CD in Appendix D) while you are waiting to go to sleep.

(Note: All I am suggesting is that you lower your sleep aid dose by half for one night of the second week only. By lowering the weekly dose by only a small amount, this should not present any problem. But it will help you build confidence that you can break the habit. If, at the first attempt, it causes a bad sleep night, you will be able to recover quickly from the next few nights' normal doses. Talk with your doctor if you have questions about this.)

4. For the third week: Add a second night when you can reduce the sleep dose by half, in addition to the other night. Don't choose two nights in succession—spread them out. Now you have lowered the dose by half for two nights of the week—say on Tuesday and Friday nights. So far, so good. Continue with your relaxation exercises.

5. For subsequent weeks: If you can tolerate the sleep aid reduction for two nights of the week, then choose an additional night and continue to lower the dose by half for the third night of the week. Then in the following week add a fourth night, and so on. Eventually you will have lowered your aid for the whole week by half. Do not try to speed up the process, as you can have a setback. The strategy is to lower the dose in small increments, then wait until your brain adapts to this reduction and starts to manufacture its own sleep aid. Then continue with the next reduction.

(Note: If you have a bad reaction at any point, go back to the last level of reduction. Hold it there for a week, then go to the next reduction.)

6. When you have lowered the dose of your sleep aid by half for every night of the week, continue by repeating the same process again. But this time you will drop the second half of the pill one night of the week, keep it there for the week, then remove the second night's doses, keep it there for a week, and so forth until you are not taking any sleeping pills at all. If at any time you have a bad reaction, go back to the previous week's level and repeat it until your brain adjusts, then continue to the next step.

Obviously, this seems like a tedious process, and it is. But it's an effective way to break your dependence on sleeping pills.

If your sleeping pill cannot be split in half, then follow the same strategy I've outlined above, but you have to double up and drop a whole pill at a time. So, for the first week, you just omit one day's sleeping pill. Then continue taking your pills for the rest of the week. Then remove the second pill, and so on. Try not to speed up the process. If you blow it, just go back to the beginning and start all over again.

Sleeping Pills and Your Kids

Is there anything more beautiful than a child fast asleep? I think not. But what a battle many parents are having today trying to get their children to sleep well! And this raises a vexing question for parents: Should they ever consider using sleeping pills for their children?

I know this battle because I felt it as a parent. There are times when you have an irresistible urge to offer something to your child to help him or her fall asleep. We have competing agendas, don't we? They want to stay awake when we want them to go to sleep. If only they came equipped with a sleep switch so that we could flick a finger and finally get that blissful, rare peace and quiet that every parent craves at the end of a long day. And then there is the struggle to keep them asleep. Midnight trips to the toilet, wanting to slip into bed with you, or nights of coughing when they have a cold. If only there was a safe, easy way to get them some sleep so we could get some sleep also!

But the bad news is that there are no safe, trouble-free ways to get children to sleep, and so the subject of sleeping pills raises many challenges. While most parents know that children should not be given sleeping pills just for the parent's convenience, should it always be avoided? There are strong feelings on both sides among experts.

You need to know that the U.S. Food and Drug Administration (FDA) has not approved any sleeping pill for use by children. "However, an estimated 180,000 Americans under the age of 20 take prescription sleep aids," according to a *New York Times* report from November 2005.[4] Furthermore, a study by Medco Health Solutions found that the "use of sleeping pills by those under age 20 has increased 85 percent since the year 2000."[5]

Adolescents, in particular, are at risk for insomnia (except on weekends), addiction, and abuse. They have trouble sleeping, whether because of stress, overstimulation, or changes in their body clock. But sleep experts are worried that sleeping pills may be over-prescribed when it comes to youth.[6]

Let's take a look at Becky, a healthy eight-year-old. She goes to bed at an appropriate time, 8:30 PM, but then lies awake until after midnight. Then the next morning, when mom goes to wake her, she can't get her out of bed. When Mom finally does get her up, she's cranky and persistently resistant. She won't get dressed; she won't eat her breakfast; and taking her to school is worse than taking her to the dentist! (With apologies to all dentists out there!) When she does get to school, she does poorly. Mom has tried everything, but Becky just can't go to sleep at bedtime, and Mom feels helpless. She has followed all the sleep rules she has heard or read about: There is no TV in her bedroom. She allows a "wind-down" time to gradually get her to bed. Becky takes a nice bath, and goes to bed consistently at the same time. Mom reads a little to her, then prays. Oh boy, does she pray! But still the problem persists. Is this a situation where a sleeping pill may be appropriate? Dilemmas like this face many parents every day.

Take another dilemma. There are developmental disorders, such as ADHD and autism, where sleep patterns are severely disturbed. Should a parent consider using a sleeping pill in these circumstances? There are no simple answers. Parents need to seek competent counsel from a sleep expert, because each situation is different.

Fortunately, there is a little ray of hope here. A recent study, using the natural hormone melatonin, was found to be effective in promoting sleep 60 percent of the time in autistic kids.[7] Melatonin, therefore, may be a safe option. But still, with only a 60 percent success rate, this won't help every child with a developmental disorder who can't sleep.

So when are sleeping pills safe for a child to use? Let me sound some warnings first, before making some recommendations. Be aware that no sleeping pill currently available has been developed specifically for use by children. Also, we just don't know what the long-term effects of sleeping pills are in children. We know that in adults the frequent use of a sleep aid makes the brain lazy. So, is it likely to be less destructive in children? I think not. There is the possibility that long-term use of sleep aids in children could create a lifelong dependence on them. And since the brains of children are still developing, it's possible that these medications could adversely affect development in ways that will cause problems throughout life.

Basically, I believe that when it comes to sleep, whether it is in adults or children, we are better off using the natural sleep mechanisms of the brain, rather than artificial aids. Only very occasionally, such as during an emergency, should one consider using a sleeping pill. Wherever possible, psychotherapeutic sleep strategies need to be followed. Also, never give your child a sleeping pill that is prescribed for you. Your doctor needs to determine the most appropriate drug and its dosage given your child's age and weight.

Here, then, are some guidelines for parents to follow when considering sleeping pills for their kids:

- The use of sleep medication should never be a physician's or parent's first choice. Some would say that it shouldn't be the second or third either! Other options, including behavioral changes, must be considered first.
- When appropriate, say where a child clearly has a disorder that can be aggravated by sleeplessness, then medications should be considered. One should start with a "natural" aid like melatonin and if necessary, in close consultation with your child's doctor, move to stronger sleep aids.
- Even if you do add a sleep medication, parents need to be diligent in making behavioral changes. These include a regular bedtime routine and setting aside adequate time for sleep. This is important because the child's use of sleeping pills is bound to make a parent less diligent in exercising sleep discipline. One leaves the pill to do all the work!
- And here also, as with adults, sleep medications should never be used on a long-term basis. The potential for developing dependence on a sleep aid is extremely high in children and teens.

11

Six Strategies That Can Help Your Family Sleep Better

*And if tonight my soul may find her peace
in sleep and sink in good oblivion,
and in the morning wake like a new-opened flower,
then I have been dipped again in God, and new-created.*
—D. H. LAWRENCE

In this chapter I will shift from explaining specific sleep habits to now summarizing six general strategies that can improve your and your family's general sleep routine. Even if you don't have a sleep problem, you will find these sleep strategies helpful in improving the overall quality of your sleep. They are designed to help you and your family fall asleep sooner and stay asleep longer.

Strategy #1
Creating a Healthy Sleep Environment

Let's start with the most basic strategy of all: ensuring that there is nothing in your environment that can rob you of precious sleep. We've touched on this before, but here I will offer a few practical, environmental basics to keep in mind:

- Make sure your sleeping environment is quiet. If you live in a noisy environment, invest in earplugs. My wife and I did that years ago, when we had neighbors with a midnight barking dog. And we have slept with them ever since. They are easy to get used to and effectively shut out a lot of extraneous noise. We sleep deeper and more peacefully if our brains don't have to block out background noises.
- Invest in a good mattress and comfortable pillows. I can't tell you how often I hear from an insomniac: "Oh, I have had the same mattress and pillows for thirty years. I've never considered that they might be so uncomfortable as to disrupt my sleep!"
- Control your room temperature. Try to maintain a comfortable temperature in your bedroom. Extreme temperatures disrupt sleep and make it difficult to fall asleep. Lean slightly toward a cooler temperature than during the daytime, as it aids sleep.
- Do not do any work, read novels, or watch TV late at night—unless the work, book, or television program is dull and boring! These will only cause your adrenal system to become aroused. If you can only fall asleep while reading or watching TV, you've conditioned your body and developed a bad habit. Start breaking the habit right away. How? Just stop allowing yourself to fall asleep in front of the TV. If you are ready for sleep, go to bed!

Strategy #2
Dealing with Your Overactive Mind

There are many occasions when bothersome thoughts rise from nowhere, possibly fed by an overactive mind, and take control of our consciousness. And nighttime seems to open the door to them. Someone has said, "If a man had as many ideas during the day as he does when he has insomnia, he'd make a fortune." Thoughts that come from an overactive mind intrude unnecessarily into your sanity and rob you of sleep, and no matter how hard you try, you cannot seem to get rid of them.

So you need to develop some strategies for untroubling and disconnecting your mind. You have to know how to force your mind away from exciting mental activities. If you must think, then learn to control your thoughts by directing them to less-activating matters. Uncontrolled thinking is a sleep killer. Following are several strategies that can help. Try each of them, then select the one that works best for you.

Thought Stopping

This technique has been used by clinicians for many years, and I've taught it to many patients with great success. Here is what you do: As you lie on your bed in a comfortable position, select a thought that sometimes bothers you. Let's say it is something about your boss that aggravates you. Take a deep, abdominal breath (push your stomach out, not in) and let the air out slowly. Relax every part of your body. Remind yourself of the troublesome thought (you might have forgotten it by now). Then snap your fingers and say "stop" to yourself. Then take a deep abdominal breath and relax again. The thought will try to come back again, and if it does, repeat the finger snap and say the word "stop" again. If it returns, say "stop," repeating it with the snaps. Later when you have conditioned the word "stop" to the finger snap, you can just think the word in your mind and it will have the same effect.

Thought Redirecting

It isn't always easy to just stop thinking about something, and many find it near impossible when their minds are just too active. So, here is a modification. It is based on the principle that it is easier to redirect your thoughts, that is, to shift the focus of your thinking elsewhere, than to stop them. For instance, let's suppose you have a work colleague who is bothering you. During your coffee break one day he says something that annoys you. That night as you try to go to sleep you catch yourself dwelling on your colleague's remarks. You can't stop them from playing like a broken record in your head. Here is how you proceed:

Relax in your bed and intentionally remind yourself of the troublesome comments. Say "stop" silently to yourself as in the previous exercise, then immediately begin to think about your colleague. Visualize his office or workplace, his desk, the machine he works with, and then try to think of a few good things you know about him. Is he a good father? Can he tell a funny joke? Try as best you can to come up with something positive he has said to you in the past. If you find nothing good to recall, think about his wife and children. Think about how human he is—no better than you, but also no worse. And so on, and so on . . . The basic strategy here is to substitute a chain of thoughts that originate with the bothersome one, but which slowly take you away from them to something more positive and pleasant.

By redirecting your thinking away from the original bothersome thought, you allow your mind to be active, but now with more wholesome, healthy, and healing thoughts. The Christian can focus this redirection ultimately on Christ, His love for us, His glorious salvation, and His call for us to forgive those who offend us, just as He has forgiven us. This always sobers me up! And there are always a lot of positive things for you to think about, so try to redirect your thinking. It takes a little practice, but once you master this technique it can become a very healthy habit!

Thought Substitution

This is the one that works best for me. Thought substitution is a refinement of thought redirecting. It differs in that you deliberately plan ahead to have three or four "thought projects" available to substitute for the troublesome thought. By thought projects I mean ideas, plans, conquests, or dreams that excite you and can captivate your mind. It can be a replay of something you did on vacation, or a place you visited. We all have things we want to do; build, plan, create—or just imagine. If you can substitute one of these interesting, but less troublesome thoughts, you should be able to distract your mind from the bothersome thought. I do it often and it is very effective.

To illustrate, let me give you an example of one of my own thought projects. I once learned to fly an airplane. Often when trying to go to sleep I will rehearse the flying exercises I had been taught—in my imagination. This is good practice and helps me to remember the complex tasks of flying. And then I discovered that if something was bothering me, I merely had to start thinking about one of my flying routines, and my mind gave up on the troublesome thoughts. It is an effective way of blocking out unwanted thoughts. Even though I no longer fly, I still enjoy rehearsing the exercise in my mind. It brings back pleasant memories of flying high above the fields of South Africa, and even though I am just lying in bed, I can still spend a few minutes flying in my imagination—and enjoying every minute of it.

Here is how you should proceed: Prepare by making a short list of suitable projects or memories that excite you. It doesn't matter if they are only imaginary. Examples could be designing a dress, planning a vacation, reliving a travel trip, going to the beach or the mountains, reciting Scripture, preaching a sermon, writing a book, or just creating and telling yourself a story. There is no limit to the "thought projects" you can invent for your mind.

These projects are then substituted the moment you have said "stop" to an unwanted thought. You redirect your thinking toward one of these projects and continue to think about it as long as it is necessary to distract yourself from the bothersome thought. If the first thought project you try doesn't do the trick, try the next. The secret is to have several of these projects up your sleeve and ready to go at a moment's notice. It helps to write down the titles of these thought projects on a card and have it ready to use.

Strategy #3
Overcoming Sleep Anxiety

Anxiety, especially worry proneness, also activates your mind. Unfortunately, worriers easily become chronic insomniacs. Going to bed seems to open every anxiety door in your mind. Invariably, those who are anxious about many things also worry about not being able to get to sleep. So if you are prone to anxiety, you should master a strategy for coping with it. (If you have a more serious problem, I recommend that you read my book *The Anxiety Cure*.[1])

The simple strategy I will present here works with most forms of worry anxiety. Breaking the worry habit can be accomplished if you do not try to cut it off. The more you fight worry, the more it fights back. Early in my career I learned a technique for dealing with worry that I would like to share here. I don't recall who came up with the idea or if any research has ever validated the method, but I have used it so often with so many patients that I know it is effective in most. In this strategy you invite the worry into your mind—and then prolong the worry as long as possible. Yes, I know this sounds ridiculous and is certainly paradoxical, but it works.

The idea behind it is that if you have short periods of worrying, say for between three and ten minutes, you tend to "incubate" your worry. That is, it is reinforced. However, if you deliberately worry about something for longer than this, the paradoxical effect is that your mind gets tired of worrying and gives up on it—effectively extinguishing the worry habit. It is in this "middle" range of worrying that worry habits are maintained. This explains why worry tends to "feed on itself."

To put it another way, we don't worry continuously even if we are chronic worriers. We worry for short periods, with breaks in between. If we did worry continuously, we would probably extinguish it. Nor do we tend to worry for just a brief period and then set it aside. This would also extinguish the worry. Instead we worry long enough to entrench our anxious feelings, and then we leave our worry alone for a while so it can "incubate" and come back to haunt us again at some other time. It is this pattern that makes worrying so resistant to extinction.

So if you are a pre-sleep worrier, here is the strategy I recommend:

- Deliberately set aside some "thinking time" for worrying as you lie down in bed. If possible, keep a notepad and pen next to you. My wife has a notepad with an attached light, and this is perfect because you can stay in bed, not bother your spouse, and make copious notes.

- Write down, briefly, what it is that is bothering you. Just a short, cryptic phrase will do, not a long essay. Writing it down is important because it helps you if you externalize the worry. Putting it down on paper tells your brain that you know what's bothering you, so it can let go of it. For instance, let's imagine you have a job interview or a doctor's appointment tomorrow that is bothering you. Write down "Interview with . . ." or "See Dr. . . . tomorrow." Believe me, by externalizing your worry (writing it on paper so you can see it), you're helping your brain to stop reminding you of it over and over again. It's there right on the paper for the world to see.

- Now notice the time on your night clock. Close your eyes and deliberately start to worry about the interview or appointment that's on your notepad. Focus on it. Think about it. If your mind tries to go somewhere else (it will definitely try to do this), pull it back. And try to keep the worry going for more than 10 minutes.

• It is very likely that along the way your mind wants to wander somewhere else long before the 10 minutes are up, and if it does not come back to the worry topic, so be it. Let it go and get to sleep. If it comes back, repeat the process. You are training a critical part of your brain (called the amygdala) to not treat the topic of your worry as something dangerous.

The main point to keep in mind here is that intentional worrying de-conditions the part of the brain that causes the worrying. When you intentionally think about something, you are telling your brain that there is nothing really threatening here—so let it go. With a little practice, you will get the idea and discover how effective it is.

Strategy #4
Collaborating with Your Melatonin System

As explained earlier in the book, the pineal gland in the brain starts to produce melatonin when darkness sets in. It is a system that works in harmony with nature's sunrises and sunsets, and sets your brain's diurnal clock. But in modern times, the system struggles to function properly because we have prolonged daylight into the late hours of the night. If you understand how the melatonin system works, it is quite easy to take control of it and manage it to your advantage. It's all about balancing light and darkness.

The average American adult only gets about one hour of natural sunlight a day. People work in factories or offices that offer little direct sunlight, and when we go home we sit in artificially lit houses. Even the best of artificial light doesn't match sunlight. This deficiency in sunlight exposure affects our circadian rhythm and is not enough to establish healthy sleep rhythm patterns. Then all you need is for it to get cloudy and you are definitely not getting enough sunlight to effectively control your melatonin system.

Here is how to manage your natural melatonin:

- First, engage in outdoor activities as much as possible during the day. At the end of the day, take the kids for a hike while there is still sunlight. If you want to sit, sit outside. The more light exposure you and your family can get during the day, the better. I don't mean direct sunlight, as in sunbathing or going hatless, but your eyes must see bright, sun-based light, not fluorescent look-alike light that masquerades for the real thing.

- Then when it gets dark, embrace the darkness. Our homes are too brightly lit for our sleep's good. So here is the rule: Darken your home environment at least one hour before you go to bed. Darkening your home jump-starts the sleepiness that is a necessary transition to sleep. My wife and I do this by having night-lights scattered about our home, giving us, and our dog, enough light to get around safely. And as soon as dinner is over, we turn off our bright lights and the night-lights take over. It is quite amazing how well you can see when your eyes adapt to some darkness. Reading with a lamp or watching TV at a distance is fine, as these are not bright enough to affect melatonin production.

- If you waken during the night, don't turn on the light and get up unless you absolutely must. If you have a bladder or prostate problem and must "get up and go," install low-level night-lights. Your goal should be to keep your melatonin flowing all through the night.

Strategy #5
Embracing Relaxation and Meditation Techniques

I have mentioned several times the importance of knowing some relaxation exercises. My *Relaxation and Christian Meditation* CD, described in Appendix D, covers a number of relaxation exercises that can facilitate sleep onset.

Here is how you should proceed:

- At bedtime, or after a nighttime awakening, choose one of the exercises. Different moods need different exercises. Don't get out of bed or go to another room. You want to associate relaxation with sleeping.

- Be realistic. Relaxation, as good as it is, is not a magic sleeping pill. So do not expect the relaxation techniques themselves to induce sleep every night. What they do is lower your arousal level. If the technique you are using doesn't help after a few nights, switch to one of the others.

- Watch your breathing. Controlling your breathing is an essential part of relaxation. And it is good for beginners because breathing is a natural function. Mostly it occurs autonomically (you don't have to think about it), but taking control of it helps you to focus away from troubling distractions and ensures that you are doing breathing that is relaxing, not tension producing.

  Many make the mistake of breathing with their chest instead of their diaphragm. Chest breathing, raising and lowering your chest when you breathe, is shallow and not relaxing. In diaphragmatic breathing the technique is to raise and lower your stomach because this pulls down your diaphragm and gives a deeper breath. One way to ensure that you are doing it right is to place your hand on the center of your stomach, just below your rib cage. Then as you breathe in, make sure your hand and stomach are moving out from your body—as if reaching for the sky. In chest breathing you pull in your stomach, and this makes for shallow breathing.

• Scan your body as you relax. Focus attention on different parts of your body and see if any part feels tenser than the rest. Become aware of your body's various sensations, whether it's pain, tension, warmth, or relaxation.

In addition to relaxation, meditation can also be a valuable aid to sleep. Not only does it facilitate relaxation and a lowering of your arousal level, but meditating on thoughts that are uplifting can benefit you spiritually and psychologically. Meditation also activates the most thoughtful part of your brain, called the "pre-frontal cortex," according to Dr. Daniel Amen, a neuro-psychiatrist.[2]

Many devout Christians associate meditation only with Eastern religions. But meditation is also a part of our Christian heritage. It's just unfortunate that we have ignored it for so long that many have come to think of it as exclusively the domain of other religions and shied away from it. I believe that this has been to our detriment. Since meditation is as much a Christian spiritual practice as anyone else's, I will discuss it more fully in the final chapter.

Strategy #6
Creating a "Sleep Aid Package"

To help you prepare yourself and your family for better sleep, you need to put together a "sleep aid package" for each of you, tailored to your ages, and have it readily available at each of your bedsides. Many hotels now offer such a package to travelers, and if they are helpful for travelers, then there is no reason why they cannot be helpful for families as well. The package I propose here, I hope, offers a few extra sleep goodies. Encourage your family to take their sleep packages with them when they travel—on business trips, going to summer camp, or on a family vacation. These trips away from home can be very sleep disruptive, so the help a sleep package gives can be a blessing.

The list of items I suggest, described in detail in Appendix C, can serve as your shopping list. Here is a brief description of what it should include, and why:

- **Eye mask.** This helps to achieve a constant state of darkness, no matter where you are, so your melatonin won't be interrupted. Such a cover for your eyes is also necessary during the summertime when morning comes early and brings light into your bedroom prematurely, or when you are traveling and your hotel room is not totally dark. Even in cross-country flying, while the plane's lights are turned off so you can sleep, there is always someone who has insomnia and insists on having his reading light on. He usually sits next to me—or you!

- **Earplugs.** Just as eye covers help to keep darkness constant, so earplugs can help you create a background sound constancy. I started using earplugs 25 years ago, and they have revolutionized my sleep quality. No matter where I am, in my bed at home or in a hotel, my background noise is always the same—quiet! I get many letters from conference attendees who thank me for emphasizing the value of earplugs.

- **Night-light.** A night-light (can be a small flashlight or a low-level wall light) is helpful both at home and on the road. We put a wall light in the bathroom wall plug so we can see our way there in the dark. It provides a soft light during the night so we can get up without turning on the main light.

- **Some sort of aroma spray.** Not only do your ears and eyes adjust to a certain constant background when you sleep, but your nose does too. Your bedroom should have a familiar smell, say by occasionally releasing lavender or another nice-smelling fragrance. By bringing the same aroma to your hotel room, you create a familiarity that can prompt sleep. After all, we go to a lot of trouble having the right aroma in our cars after a car wash, so why not also in the bedroom?

So this is a basic Sleep Aid Package. You may have a few other comforts of your own to add, such as a soft music player. When traveling, I usually add a packet of antacids and a mild painkiller in case I get a headache from the travel. Keep it right next to your bed within easy reach. Also make a Sleep Aid Package for each member of your family so they don't come and steal yours! It makes a great birthday or Christmas gift and reminds everyone that sleeping well is the road to a fulfilling and happy life.

12

Sleep and Your Family's Spirituality

Of all the thoughts of God that are borne inward unto souls afar,
along the Psalmist's music deep,
now tell me if that any is for gift or grace, surpassing this—
"He giveth His beloved sleep."
—ELIZABETH BARRETT BROWNING, "THE SLEEP"

And the peace of God, which transcends all understanding,
will guard your hearts and your minds in Christ Jesus.
—PHILIPPIANS 4:7

Up to this point, I have refrained from making too many comments about how our sleep is related to the spiritual side of our lives. Some readers may not have any interest in this, but for those who do, this chapter addresses how sleep is important to building a healthy spirituality. Because I am a Christian, my focus here will be primarily on Christian spiritual practices, but I hope that what I have to say will be beneficial to those of other faiths as well. For me, the part of my day that makes me feel closest to God is my pre-sleep time. No intrusions or distractions. Nothing waiting for my attention. Just me and my God.

But what has this got to do with families? A lot. For starters, what Mom and Dad believe about sleep and its spiritual connection will most certainly influence what they teach their children. But more importantly, if healthy sleep can shape a healthy spirituality, then it is most imperative that we have a clear understanding of what spiritual disciplines and practices can revolve around good sleep. In short, it does a family good!

Sleep Is Important to the Soul

Unfortunately, I don't think I've ever heard a sermon on sleep. Have you? Take a look at Scottish theologian John Baillie's writing in his famous work *Christian Devotion*:

> My subject is the theology of sleep. It is an unusual subject, but I make no apology for it. I think we hear too few sermons about sleep. After all, we spend a very large share or our lives sleeping. . . . Don't you agree that the Christian gospel should have something to say about the sleeping third of our lives as well as about the waking two-thirds of it?[1]

Yes, I do agree. There is something incredibly spiritual about sleep—for us as well as for our families. Fulfilling sleep is the gateway to an exquisite, sublime state of serenity—a wondrous peacefulness that only God can give! It allows us to transcend our wakeful world and break free from earth's limitations; to step out of the shackles of real life and experience an amazing sort of freedom, if only for a short while.

One liberating sleep experience my wife loves comes in a frequent dream. In this dream she flies like a bird, or should I say, like an angel. At least that's how she describes it. Soaring into the sky, she feels no gravity. She can fly anywhere, just like the angels. It is her favorite dream and always leaves her feeling renewed. Unfortunately, my flying dreams always end with the feeling that I am dropping out of the sky, in free fall, with nothing to prevent me from crashing into the ground!

Your Pre-Sleep Pondering

While I have no doubt that sleeping well can enhance your spiritual experiences and that the lack of sleep can undermine your spirituality, I can't help feeling that what is most important is the short period that precedes our actual falling asleep—our pre-sleep preparation. This is where the really important link between sleep and spirituality occurs, in you and in members of your family. In other words, while sleep is important in restoring our brain to healthy functioning, our pre-sleep period may be even more important spiritually. It's what we do in our thinking and reflecting in those last minutes, and sometimes hours, before falling into oblivion that influences the sleep that follows. And if God is a part of it, He will also be a part of what follows.

It is important that I reflect briefly on the theology of sleep. There is a most illuminating verse in Psalm 4, sometimes referred to as one of the "sleep psalms," that is most relevant here. I'm very aware of the dangers in taking Scripture words too literally, but see if you find this verse relevant: "I will lie down and sleep in peace" (v. 8).

But in an earlier verse, the psalmist had said, "When you are on your beds, search your hearts and be silent" (v. 4). The words "search your hearts" have also been translated as "ponder in your hearts."

True, the context here is about being angry when you go to bed. But I think it has a much broader implication. In effect, this verse tells us that *sleeping peacefully depends on what you ponder in your silence before going to sleep.* Don't you think this would make a great poster to hang above your bed? It could certainly have a profound effect on the quality of your and your family's sleep.

Not a lot of research has been done into the benefits of our pre-sleep period. Mostly, research here has focused on finding ways to speed up sleep onset, say with imagery techniques. My intention in this last chapter is not to speed up the onset of sleep, but to utilize this valuable time to enhance spiritual practices. However, from my experience, the exercises I will describe do help sleep onset, simply because they are designed to create a peaceful mindset.

So in this final chapter, I will focus on the pre-sleep period—King David's "pondering in silence before you go to sleep." Hopefully, we can find ways to turn our sleep into a daily experience of God, or as someone else has described it, "a restored wholeness."

Christian Myths That Can Undermine Sleep

But before setting out some practical pre-sleep exercises, I need to briefly address two misconceptions that, in my experience in counseling, can undermine healthy sleep habits.

First, many Christians I encounter firmly believe good sleeping habits do not facilitate a vibrant spirituality. I have had many Christians in my seminars interject comments such as, "The Bible doesn't endorse sleep. It calls the sleepy person slothful"—referring to a verse such as Proverbs 6:9: "How long wilt thou sleep, O sluggard? when wilt thou arise out of thy sleep?" (KJV).

I also know many pastors who believe that somehow, because they "do God's work," they are exempt from the laws of His nature, especially as it relates to sleep. "I've got God's work to do. I can't waste my time sleeping the day away." How wrong they are. Jesus had the most incredible mission to accomplish, but He certainly found time for sleep and rest. Matthew 8:23–27 tells of how Jesus even slept on a boat on the sea during a great storm, and there are several times when He was tired and rested, such as sitting on the wall of a well when the adulterous woman approached to fetch water. He often encouraged His disciples to take their rest.

Second, there is another complicating factor. Many Christians go so far as to hold the misleading belief that sleep and God's kingdom don't mix. In other words, to be a godly person you have to deprive yourself of sleep, not try to get more. Building spiritual disciplines takes time, and this means less sleep, not more. From this perspective, too much sleep is seen as destructive to your soul, and it doesn't build God's kingdom. They would assert that "you are just wasting God's time, time that you should be spending on saving souls or feeding the poor." A pastor friend of mine once told me that his basic life philosophy was to accomplish as much as he possibly could in this life. Then he added, "I'll have lots of time to sleep when I am dead." Two months later, he suffered a heart attack and died.

I wonder how Jesus would respond to such a philosophy. He fell asleep in the back of a boat once, and it nearly sank because of a terrible storm. I can picture Him lying peacefully (on a cushion, Scripture tells us) during that furious storm. He was so at peace that He had to be awakened by His disciples because they feared they would all perish (Mark 4:38). Why would He sleep during a dangerous storm? And why, knowing that His life was going to be short, would He sleep when people needed rescuing? The incarnate Jesus, who had taken upon Himself a human body, must have thought that sleep was important.

Many also use Scripture, like Matthew 26:36–46, to reinforce their belief that you can sleep too much. This passage describes Jesus in the Garden of Gethsemane telling His disciples to "stay here and keep watch" over Him as He goes off to pray alone. But when He returns He finds them sleeping. So He chastises them with: "Could you men not keep watch with me for one hour? Watch and pray so that you will not fall into temptation. The spirit is willing, but the body is weak."

Then He goes away again, but when He returns He finds them sleeping again "because their eyes were heavy." Returning a third time, He says to them: "Are you still sleeping and resting? . . . Rise, let us go! Here comes my betrayer!"

Let me be clear that scriptures like this were not intended to keep us away from sleep. In biblical times, as in the ancient world, insomnia as we know it today was relatively non-existent.[2] Sure, people may have had an occasional sleepless night, but not for want of being able to sleep. And they could always count on plenty of sleep time to make up for what was lost. Troubling circumstances demanded wakefulness, but once the trouble was over, sleep naturally returned.

There are times when sleep has to be sidelined. I can clearly recall such an occasion that robbed me of sleep in my own early adulthood. My wife and I, newly married, were spending a holiday with my grandfather. He was retired and had a small farm out in the country on the banks of the great Vaal River in South Africa, growing vegetables and raising chickens. Our visit coincided with hatching time—when the eggs for the next year's crop of chickens were being hatched in a large incubator my grandfather had built. Late one cold night, right after going to bed, there was a terrible rainstorm. Strong winds and lightning pulled down the power lines serving the area so the chicken incubators that used electric heaters went cold, and part of the roof over the chicken breeding area was blown off. Many hundreds of newly born chicks were at risk of dying.

This was not a time for sleep. We all jumped out of bed and rallied to rescue the chicks, drying them and trying to keep them warm by whatever means possible. Imagine my wife and me cuddling hundreds of chickens in front of the quickly lit fireplace, trying to warm them with our own bodies.

It was a long night, but by daybreak we had salvaged most of the chicks and set up pens for them on the back veranda. Exhausted, we went to bed for a little sleep. That was a night when sleep was out of the question—and your body understands it in a remarkable way, mobilizing the resources built into us for such emergencies.

Yes, there are times when we should be chastised for sleeping when we should be "keeping a lookout" or dealing with an emergency. But this is not the same as the perpetual over-arousal that we experience in our modern-day lifestyle. We are not called to live a life that is deficient in sleep just so we can be more spiritual. In biblical times, people didn't have the sleep disruptions from which we suffer today. No late-night TV or Internet games. Darkness prevailed, and with it came deep sleep. There may have been times of crisis that required people to over-ride their need for sleep so as to deal with the crisis, but this is hardly justification for abandoning all sleep in ordinary times.

Letting Go of Wakefulness

The point I am building up to here is this: You can turn sleep and spirituality into compatible bed-fellows that can be stress relieving and spirit enhancing. Charles Spurgeon, the great British preacher of the mid-1800s, once preached a sermon on the text "When thou liest down, thou shalt not be afraid: yea, thou shalt lie down, and thy sleep shall be sweet" (Proverbs 3:24, KJV). This is what he said:[3]

> When we go to bed at night, let this word smooth our pillow.
> We cannot guard ourselves in sleep, but the Lord will keep us
> through the night. Those who lie down under the protection of
> the Lord are as secure as kings and queens in their palaces, and a
> great deal more so. If with our lying down there is a laying down
> of all cares and ambitions, we shall get refreshment out of our
> beds such as the anxious and covetous never find in theirs. Ill
> dreams shall be banished, or even if they come, we shall wipe
> out the impression of them, knowing that they are only dreams.

So, to help you "lay down all cares and ambitions," here are some spiritual practices that can turn your pre-sleep time into a deeply spiritual experience. And at the same time you will be able to "lie down and sleep in peace" (Psalm 4:8). Most of them can be adapted for your children as well.

Centering Yourself

Make it your first priority, when going to bed, to focus and center back on yourself. Most of us live fragmented lives, rushing here and there throughout every day. We feel overwhelmed by life's many demands, and invariably end each day with the feeling that we have not accomplished all we wanted to. One person recently described her end-of-day feelings as "dotty, disorderly, and disjointed." An apt alliteration! She went on to say, "One part of me seems to be going north, another part south, and the rest down a big hole like Alice in Wonderland; except there's nothing wonderful in the land!"

What happens is that a sort of depersonalization overtakes us when we are rushed, pushed, and pulled, with no time to collect our thoughts. We feel like puppets, jumping to the strings of others. The more we are pressured, the more vague and dreamlike our world feels. We feel detached from ourselves, as if we are outsiders looking in, rather than being at the center of our lives.

This is not a good state of mind for sleep. For one thing, it leaves your brain confused. Remember, while you sleep the brain has work to do, consolidating, clarifying, healing, and growing new connections. So the more centered you are—with a feeling that you are in control and at the center of your life, not just an observer—the better.

One exercise espoused by those who follow a contemplative spirituality is to use a "centering prayer," a prayer that places a strong emphasis on interior silence. The roots of such a prayer go back to the early days of Christianity, but we are now seeing a revival of interest in contemplative spiritual practices, as many Protestants have begun to espouse these as styles of worship and personal devotion.

The purpose of a centering prayer is to help you clear your mind of intrusive thoughts so that you can focus on the presence of God. One well-known centering prayer is called "The Jesus Prayer." It is a short prayer in which the words "Lord Jesus Christ, Son of God, have mercy on me, a sinner" are repeated.

Now, you don't have to follow anyone else here. You can create your own centering prayer. Here are some suggestions; adapt them to your prayer style:

- As you lie comfortably in bed with your eyes closed, relax and quiet yourself. Slow down your thinking. Try to focus on this as a time of prayer.
- Reflect for a moment on how loving God is—to you, to your family, and to the world.
- Choose a word or phrase of Scripture that you find comforting and that best supports your sincere intention to be in the Lord's presence (e.g., "Jesus," "Lord," "God," "Savior," "Shalom," "Spirit," "Love," and so on). My favorite is the phrase "God's peace."
- Keep this word or phrase present in your mind. Repeat it slowly, over and over.
- Whenever you are distracted, return to your scriptural phrase, as if it is an anchor. After a short while, continue with the next exercise.

For children, centering can take the form of a conversation. Have your children share a story with you about something that has happened during the day. Is anything bothering them? Are they excited about tomorrow? Your goal here is to try to resolve any intrusive thoughts and help your children lay them aside. Then as you pray with them, make your prayer a centering prayer as well. Is there a special Scripture verse they would like you to recite? I clearly remember that when my brother and I stayed with my grandparents during school holidays, my grandmother would ask me, the older, to choose a verse from the Bible and read it aloud for all of us.

Pre-Sleep Meditation

The Psalms are full of references to meditating on God. Psalm 1:1–2 says, "Blessed is the man . . . [whose] delight is in the law of the LORD, and on his law he meditates day and night." Psalm 19:14 declares, "May the words of my mouth and the meditation of my heart be pleasing in your sight, O LORD, my Rock and my Redeemer."

We need to embrace stillness and silence at some point in our day. The end of the day, just before going to sleep, is the perfect time. As I write this, I am in Hawaii, speaking at a combined church conference. Reading the newspaper this morning, I came across several announcements of meditation workshops being offered by local churches. One was called "Learning to be still and quiet." Another, "The value of silent prayer." And one church offered "A quiet morning from 9 AM to 11:30 AM" each day of the week, where you can just slip into the church for a time of stillness—and stay as long as you like. I hope it's not just Hawaii that appreciates the value of stillness!

Now, I realize that many cannot take a morning off to go and experience stillness and quietness at a local church. After all, someone has to put food on the table, get the kids to school, clean the house—and on and on. So meditation time might look different for you than it does for me. But for busy people, often, the only moment in time you can embrace meditation may be the time before bed. It will certainly help you get to sleep and will even more certainly improve the quality of your sleep.

There are two essential ingredients you need to focus on as you develop the practice of Christian meditation:

1. First you must develop your ability to focus on something specific—and stay focused. Type A personalities, like myself, are all over the place in our thoughts. Thoughts flood my thinking and jump from pillar to post. Clinically, we call this "polyphasic" thinking—and I know it well and suffer from it big-time. Some of us, therefore, require disci-

plined practice so as to become "monophasic" thinkers—where you only tolerate one thought at a time. Then, and only then, is deep meditative reflection possible.

2. Second, you have to accept that worship goes beyond what you do in church. This seems obvious, I know, but my experience with many Christians is that they think that worship happens only in a church. They have never stood on the edge of a magnificent canyon or marveled at a beautiful sunset, and felt compelled to fall on their knees in an act of worship to the Creator. They have never looked into the face of a newborn baby and wanted to bless the name of the Lord. It never even dawns on them that worship can be experienced anywhere, at any moment of any day.

The Relaxation CD I offer in Appendix D also includes a section on Christian meditation with a booklet that guides you through these exercises, so I will not go into much detail here. Many of these exercises can also be adapted for your children—though my experience has been that children and teens today rarely have patience for meditation. As you design your own pre-sleep meditation, however, try to incorporate the following:

- Intentionally "let go" or surrender these moments to God. Imagine that Jesus is with you, watching over you—because He is!
- Be still; be quiet. Practice focusing on God. Imagine Him inviting you to hand over your tensions and worries. Your thoughts may wander, so keep bringing them back to the main thought on your mind. Don't give up easily.
- Keep reminding yourself that God is with you. Feel His presence welcoming you, comforting you, and smiling on you.
- Use your imagination to enhance your act of surrender. The wonderful thing about surrendering to God is that you get your life back again, magnified by His power.

• Select one attribute of God and focus on it. There is a long list you can choose from: His love, compassion, grace, long-suffering, forgiveness, and holiness can all be rich resources for your imagination. Think about how you have experienced these attributes in your own life. Have you ever felt the love of God deep down in your being? Have you ever been overwhelmed with a feeling of forgiveness?

End-of-Day Exercises

The last of the spiritual exercises I want to leave with you is a series of end-of-day exercises. If you try doing just one of them at a time for a few weeks, you will discover which of them suits your temperament best. The best time to do them is just before going to bed, or after you are in bed. What is important is that you do them before you fall asleep. There are three:

1. Fostering end-of-day gratitude
2. Forgoing end-of-day grudges
3. Focusing the end of day on God

These exercises are well received by children when parents turn it into a game of sorts. For instance, fostering end-of-day gratitude is a game the whole family can play. Merely hand out blank cards to all the family at the children's bedtime and have them do the exercise as a group, writing (or you write for them if they are too young) their answers to the games that follow. Then collect and keep the cards so you can all review them at a later time. The idea, basically, is to instill the habit of gratitude and to make it a lifelong habit.

Fostering End-of-Day Gratitude

Well-known psychologist Dr. Martin Seligman, the founder of the Positive Psychology movement that is revolutionizing the field of psychol-

ogy today, says that gratitude-building exercises can increase contentment because they can change your brain's memory and perception of
the past. Since your brain continues to process the day's activities, even
as you go to sleep, you can build a healthier mind by giving it healthier
material to work with in the closing moments of consciousness.

Though modern psychology has just discovered this idea, there is
nothing new about it. The apostle Paul advocates the exact same principle in Philippians 4:8: "Whatever is true, . . . noble, . . . right, . . . pure, . . .
lovely, . . . admirable, . . . excellent or praiseworthy—think about such
things." He understood a principle that has taken eons for psychology to
discover—how thoughts can profoundly influence your life for good. You
literally put them into practice (v. 9). Dr. Seligman introduced a strategy
for doing this that has now become a popular idea in psychotherapy. He
calls it "The Three Blessings" exercise, and it goes like this:

Every night before you go to sleep, think about three things that
went well or were blessings for you that day. In other words, what three
things happened in your day for which you are thankful? Write them
down so you can put them in your memory. Then take a few minutes
to contemplate these blessings. Seligman's research shows that they can
eclipse the bad things that might have happened to you during the day.
People who do this exercise regularly are less depressed and happier. My
guess is that they also sleep better!

For example, let's say you visited your physician for your annual
physical today. It's always an anxious time for you. *But*, everything
checked out healthy—so here is something for which to be thankful.
Or maybe you met an old friend in the waiting room whom you had not
seen for years, and renewed your acquaintance. You had been feeling
quite guilty for not having made contact over the last few years and
thought that your friend might be angry with you. But she was friendly
and now all is resolved. Chalk up another blessing.

In addition to being grateful by identifying three blessings, also identify the best moment of your day. Relive that moment in your imagination and savor the joy over again.

Here again, research has shown that savoring events in your life like
this increases your brain's awareness of pleasure and makes the pleasure
last and even become more intense.

Now, I realize that there are days when it's difficult to come up with
something for which you feel thankful. I had such a day yesterday, but
as I was lying awake at bedtime, I began my end-of-day gratitude game.
I lay there for a while, but could not for the life of me come up with a
single thing for which I was grateful. It seemed as if it were easier to
come up with a bunch of curses, not blessings. First, early in the morning a nephew from South Africa called to tell me that my brother, a
retired widower living in a retirement home by himself, had fallen next
to his bed at three o'clock in the morning and broken his leg; he could
not get up, so he lay there until morning when someone came to check
on him.

Then in the afternoon, I was clearing out a cupboard on our patio
when I disturbed a nest of wasps. They attacked and stung me in several places, some of which I can't even mention. I scrambled to get the
stings out, applied some anti-bacterial medication, covered my head
with a piece of netting my wife had in a cupboard, clothed myself from
toe to head, and went to take my revenge. But by evening I had several
swellings and a lot of stinging.

I tried to focus on finding three blessings. Nothing came to mind,
so I reviewed my day from the start again. I had had a phone call from
my oldest granddaughter in the morning. She had aced an examination
at college and wanted me to know that the model of a brain I had lent
her had helped her enormously in memorizing the parts of the brain. She
wanted to thank me. Okay, that could be blessing number one.

Then I remembered a phone call earlier from a man across the country who desperately needed help. After a short conversation, I was able to pinpoint his problem and refer him to a psychologist in his area who could help him. His sincere appreciation was overwhelming. Make that number two. I struggled for a while to come up with number three, and then suddenly it popped into my head. I could be thankful that my brother was recuperating, and my wasp stings were subsiding. Bingo! Number three. I don't remember anything after that. My sleep was peaceful!

Forgoing End-of-Day Grudges

The second group of end-of-day exercises involves disposing of your brain's recall of any unpleasant events of the day. Here again, we don't want to use sleep time to repair unnecessary painful memories. It's better to do it before you go to sleep.

If you genuinely have no grudges at the end of your day, you are indeed a blessed person. Most of us have some unpleasantness hanging about in our minds when we go to bed. Start by briefly identifying any grudge or grudges that still linger from your day. Perhaps it was a friend's snub, the rudeness of your boss, or a tiff with your teenage daughter. Whatever it was, make a mental note of it.

It is not healthy to stuff these hurts away or allow them to subconsciously hang around in the shadows of your mind. Honestly reflect on the grudge or hurt you feel for a brief period. Were you the innocent party? Did you contribute to the tiff? No matter. You can't fix it now, but perhaps in the morning you can determine to make amends. So put it on hold and move to the next, and hardest, step.

End your day, every day, with as much forgiveness as you can muster. "But I was the innocent one. He hurt me." No excuses please. Guilty or innocent, the mark of maturity is the ability to offer forgiveness whatever the hurt or whoever is guilty. After all, resentment is like a boomerang—it always comes back and hurts you even if it is justified.

What is forgiveness? If you have read my previous books you will know that I believe forgiveness is simply a matter of "surrendering my right to hurt you back."[4] Forgiveness is not a feeling, but an act of your will. You merely choose to do it. And when you take the initiative and forgive unconditionally, no matter your innocence, you are the beneficiary, and sleep comes more easily.

Focusing the End of Day on God

Who was the last person you thought about just before you fell asleep last night? It's a hard question, because we can never remember the last moments just before falling asleep. However, after your exercises in gratitude and forgiveness, there can be no more peaceful a thought to embrace as the last before falling asleep, than thinking about God.

How do you think about God? I suppose we all differ here. Some of us may have created a visual image of Jesus from some old painting, so He is easy to think about. Others, like me, have no real image of God in mind. I sometimes think of Him as I have seen Him in others who have always seemed godly to me—such as my Sunday school teacher when I was a child. Or I visualize the grandeur of His creation, such as the beauty of a flower I saw in my garden. Sometimes, it is just a sense of His presence; what I felt when I woke up after my heart surgery and was thankful I survived. I wanted to cry with joy.

So, whatever your image of God is, take the last moments before going to sleep and fill your mind with that image or awareness of God, and stay focused there until sleep finally arrives.

My Closing Words

It's a basic principle in cognitive psychotherapy that healthy thoughts will produce healthy behaviors and feelings. Christlike behavior begins as Christlike thinking. Love is first a thought, and later becomes a behavior and habit. Grace, peace, kindness, and long-suffering are first thoughts that God plants in our minds; then they emerge as actions and behaviors. The way you treat your children, serve your employer, or love your spouse will always begin as a thought—and only afterward become an action.

Unfortunately, many of the thoughts that rush to fill our minds in those last waking moments are, like weeds in a garden, difficult to eradicate. Deep within most of our minds are unpleasant-at-best and shameful-at-worst thoughts that have tortuous roots. And somehow they always try to assert themselves as we are trying to get to sleep. But take heart. God knows this, and by prayer and by continually filling your mind with the right thoughts, you will slowly win back your mind to health again, and your brain to a heavenly sleep.

In closing, let me leave you with this thought: While we were made to sleep, God promises that He will never sleep. Isn't that a wonderful thought? It is because He does not sleep that we can sleep in safety. So take courage in these words from the psalmist:

He . . . will neither slumber nor sleep.
The LORD watches over you—
the LORD is your shade at your right hand:
the sun will not harm you by day, nor the moon by night.
The LORD will keep you from all harm—he will watch over
    your life;
the LORD will watch over your coming and going both now
    and forevermore.
    —Psalm 121:4–8

AMEN.

Appendix A
Sleep Diary—Part One

COMPLETE IN THE MORNING

Date:	Went to bed at:	Fell asleep at:	Got out of bed at:	Woke up (times):	Feeling on waking:	Total time slept:	My sleep was disturbed by:
					Refreshed? Tired?		
					Refreshed? Tired?		
					Refreshed? Tired?		
					Refreshed? Tired?		
					Refreshed? Tired?		
					Refreshed? Tired?		
					Refreshed? Tired?		

Comments:

Appendix B
Sleep Diary—Part Two

COMPLETE IN THE EVENING BEFORE GOING TO BED

Date:	When did you drink caffeine?	What medications did you take?	When did you exercise?	What did you eat 2 hrs. before bed?	What did you do before bed?	
Comments:						

Appendix C
Assembling Your Sleep Aid Package

Go to your nearest drug store and purchase the following items that can serve as your Sleep Aid Package:

1. Eye mask (black and light proof)
2. Earplugs (the soft-gel type are the best)
3. A night-light (or small flashlight so you can get up without turning on the light)
4. An aroma spray (like lavender or whatever you find comforting and relaxing)
5. Lip balm (to prevent lips from drying out)
6. Hand cream (soothing and cooling to the skin)
7. Essential medications:
     • Painkiller (for headaches and so on)
     • Cough drops (throat dries out at night)
     • Decongestant (runny nose). However, decongestants should only be used on a short-term basis for nasal stuffiness, as they may cause insomnia in some people.
8. Clock (lit so it is visible in darkness)
9. Sleepytime tea (or other non-caffeine-based beverage to hydrate your body)
10. Music player (or iPod), with ear phones, for playing relaxing music

Appendix D
How to Order Dr. Hart's Relaxation
Training and Relaxing Sounds Audio CDs

The *Relaxation and Christian Meditation* audio CD is designed to do four things:

1. It will develop your ability to rapidly produce a deep state of muscle relaxation, called the relaxation response. This response minimizes your body's stress-arousal systems, including your adrenaline, cortisol, and other sad messengers, and maximizes your brain's happy and sedating messengers.

2. It will teach you how to warm your hands as a way of switching off your fight-or-flight response. The cold hands and cold feet phenomena are particularly prevalent in those who are stressed, and they easily trigger the adrenaline response.

3. It will teach you how to take control of your thoughts and redirect them in times of worry or high anxiety into more constructive channels. Included in this section will be training in how to "cut off" your worrying.

4. Lastly, it will provide you with ways you can enhance your sensory awareness of what is going on around you, and it offers Christian-based meditation exercises. Not only will these exercises help you to become more focused on God and His Word, but they will assist you in becoming more prayerful and conscious of God's presence.

Together, these exercises are widely accepted in the sleep research community as being helpful in enhancing sleep hygiene.

The *Relaxing Sounds* audio CD provides one hour of soft, soothing sounds you can listen to as you relax or meditate. One part of the CD provides a period of gentle wind chimes; the other, ocean wave sounds.

The *Relaxation and Christian Meditation* audio CD, with the booklet to guide the user, is available from Dr. Hart for $15, including postage.

The *Relaxing Sounds* audio CD costs $12, including postage.

To aid in shipping, write your name and address on a three-by-five-inch card or piece of paper (serves as a mailing label) and send it with your check to:

Dr. Archibald Hart
1042 Cyrus Lane
Arcadia, CA 91006

Other Helpful Resources by Dr. Hart

A Women's Guide to Overcoming Depression (written with daughter Dr. Catherine Hart Weber) (Grand Rapids, MI: Baker Publishing Group, 2007)

Helping Children Survive Divorce (Nashville: Thomas Nelson, 1997)

Safe Haven Marriage (written with daughter Dr. Sharon Hart May) (Nashville: Thomas Nelson, 2003)

Secrets of Eve (written with daughter Dr. Catherine Hart Weber) (Nashville: Thomas Nelson, 1998)

Stressed or Depressed: Teen Depression (written with Dr. Catherine Hart Weber) (Nashville: Thomas Nelson, 2005)

The Anxiety Cure (Nashville: Thomas Nelson, 2001)

The Sexual Man (Nashville: Thomas Nelson, 1995)

Unmasking Male Depression (Nashville: Thomas Nelson, 2001)

Thrilled to Death: How the Endless Pursuit of Pleasure Is Leaving Us Numb (Nashville: Thomas Nelson, 2007)

Details are available at Dr. Hart's Web site: www.hartinstitute.com.

Notes

Chapter 1

1. Report in the January 2007 issue of the *Harvard Heart Letter*, cited in "Poor Sleep Habits: Heart Disease and Sleep Apnea," Harvard Health press release, http://www.health.harvard.edu/press_releases /sleep-habits (accessed November 18, 2009).

2. Archibald D. Hart, *The Hidden Link Between Adrenaline and Stress* (Waco, TX: Word, 1986), 192.

3. National Sleep Foundation, *2005 Sleep in America Poll* (Washington, DC: National Sleep Foundation, 2005), http://www.sleepfoundation .org/sites/default/files/2005_summary_of_findings.pdf.

4. *Journal of Clinical Hypertension*, Vol. 4, no. 6.

5. Institute of Medicine, *Sleep Disorders and Sleep Deprivation: An Unmet Public Health Problem* (Washington, D.C.: National Academies Press, 2006), cited in National Academy of Sciences, Report Brief, April 2006, http://www.iom.edu/~/media/Files/Report%20 Files/2006/Sleep-Disorders-and-Sleep-Deprivation-An-Unmet-Public-Health-Problem/Sleepforweb.ashx (accessed November 18, 2009).

6. Gregory Stores, "Children's Sleep Disorders: Modern Approaches, Developmental Effects, and Children at Special Risk," *Developmental Medicine and Child Neurology* 41, no. 8 (1999): 568–73.

7. Ibid.

8. Mary Sykes Wylie, "Sleepless in America: Making It Through the Night in a Wired World," *Psychotherapy Networker* (March–April 2008): 3.

9. Data from U.S. National Highway Traffic Safety Administration, Fatal Accident Reporting System, 1986–1995, cited in Stanley Coren, "Sleep Deficit, Fatal Accidents, and the Spring Shift to Daylight Savings Time" (paper presented at INABIS conference, Canada,

1998) and "The Daylight Savings Time Switch and Increased Accidents," Newspaper.com, http://thenewspaper.com/news/03/300.asp.

10. National Commission on Sleep Disorders Research, U.S. Department of Health and Human Services, *Wake Up America: A National Sleep Alert, A Report of the National Commission on Sleep Disorders Research* (Washington, D.C.: Government Printing Office, 1993–1995).

11. Archibald D. Hart, *Thrilled to Death: How the Endless Pursuit of Pleasure Is Leaving Us Numb* (Nashville: Thomas Nelson, 2007).

12. Nancy Trejos, "Time May Be Up for Naps in Pre-K Class," *Washington Post*, March 15, 2004, http://www.washingtonpost .com/ac2/wp-dyn/A58706-2004Mar14?language=printer.

13. Study published in *Sleep*, September 1, 2007, cited in Alice Park, "Can't Sleep? Turn Off the Cell Phone!" *Time*, August 31, 2007, http://www.time.com/time/health/article/0,8599,1658 166,00.html.

Chapter 2

1. Thomas Roth, quoted in Mary Sykes Wylie, "Sleepless in America: Making It Through the Night in a Wired World," *Psychotherapy Networker* (March–April 2008): 27.

2. Cited in Daniel G. Amen, *Change Your Brain, Change Your Life* (New York: Three Rivers Press, 1999).

3. Study conducted by Sara Mednick et al., University of San Diego, cited in "Quick Nap Can Enhance Creativity," ABC-7, KGO-TV San Francisco, August 6, 2009, http://abclocal.go.com/kgo/story ?section=news/health&id=6952841 (accessed November 18, 2009).

4. Study conducted by Xavier Bertrand et al., French Ministry of Health and Solidarity, cited in Eva Cahen, "French Consider Benefits of Napping at Work," *CNS News*, March 2, 2007, http://www.cnsnews.com/news/print/18224.

Chapter 3

1. Calvin S. Hall, *The Meaning of Dreams* (New York: Harper, 1953).
2. Rosalind Cartwright, quoted in "Dream Research: The Sleeper Field," *Time*, August 1988, 39.
3. 2009 study conducted by the Sleep and Neuroimaging Laboratory, Department of Psychology, University of California, Berkeley, cited in Leslie Stahl, "The Science of Sleep," *60 Minutes*, March 13, 2008, documentary, http://www.cbsnews.com/stories/2008/03/14/60 minutes/main3939721.shtml (accessed November 18, 2009).

Chapter 4

1. Study conducted by Dr. Angela Clow et al., University of Westminster, London, cited in Keith Rockmael, "Sleep Away Your Stress," *MyPrimetime*, http://www.myprimetime.com/health/ailments _answers/content/sleeping_in/index.shtml (accessed November 18, 2009).
2. Archibald D. Hart, *The Anxiety Cure* (Nashville: Thomas Nelson, 2001).
3. Michael Price, "Caffeine's Wake-Up Call," *Monitor on Psychology* 39, no. 4 (2008): 26, http://www.apa.org/monitor/2008/04/caffeine.html.
4. Roland Griffiths, quoted in Price, "Caffeine's Wake-Up Call," 27.
5. D. Heseltine and J. F. Potter, "Postprandial Hypotension in Elderly People," *Age and Ageing* 19, no. 4 (1990): 233–35.
6. Information adapted from R. R. Griffiths, L. M. Juliano, and A. L. Chausmer, "Caffeine Pharmacology and Clinical Effects," in A. W. Graham et al., eds., *Principles of Addiction Medicine*, 3rd ed. (Chevy Chase, MD: American Society of Addiction, 2003), 193–224, cited in Johns Hopkins Bayview Medical Center, "Information About Caffeine Dependence," http://www.caffeinedependence.org /caffeine_dependence.html#reference1.
7. Study published in *Sleep*, http://medscape.com/viewarticle/572603.

8. Archibald D. Hart, *Unmasking Male Depression* (Nashville, Thomas Nelson, 2001) and *Unveiling Depression in Women* (Grand Rapids: Baker, 2001). Details can be found at www.hartinstitute.com.

9. Marcela Gaviria, "The Medicated Child," *Frontline*, PBS, January 8, 2008, documentary, http://www.pbs.org/wgbh/pages/frontline /medicatedchild.

Chapter 5

1. Michael J. Sateia et al., "Evaluation of Chronic Insomnia," American Academy of Sleep Medicine, cited in *Sleep* 23, no. 2 (2000): 243–308, http://www.aasmnet.org/Resources/PracticeParameters/Review_ ChronicInsomnia.pdf.

2. 1998 National Sleep Foundation "Women and Sleep" poll, cited in "Women and Sleep," National Sleep Foundation, http://www .sleepfoundation.org/article/sleep-topics/women-and-sleep (accessed November 19, 2009).

3. Study cited in Archibald D. Hart and Catherine Hart Weber, *Secrets of Eve* (Nashville: Thomas Nelson, 1998).

Chapter 6

1. Naresh M. Punjabi et al., "Sleep-Disordered Breathing and Mortality: A Prospective Cohort Study," *PLoS Medicine* 6, no. 8 (2009): http://www.plosmedicine.org/article/info:doi%2F10.1371%2F journal.pmed.1000132.

2. Seung-Schik Yoo et al., "The Human Emotional Brain Without Sleep: A Prefrontal Amygdala Disconnect," *Current Biology* 17, no. 20 (2007): 877–78, http://www.cell.com/current-biology/abstract /S0960-9822(07)01783-6.

3. Joan L. Luby et al., "Preschool Depression: Homotypic Continuity and Course over Twenty-Four Months," *Archives of General Psychiatry* 66, no. 8 (August 2009): 897–905, cited in Associated Press,

"Study: Major Depression Can Be 'Chronic' in Children as Young as Three," FoxNews.com, August 3, 2009, http://www.foxnews.com /story/0,2933,536382,00.html.

4. *National College Health Assessment: Reference Group Report* (Baltimore: American College Health Association, 2004), cited in Richard Kadison, "Getting an Edge: Use of Stimulants and Antidepressants in College," *New England Journal of Medicine* 353, no. 11 (September 15, 2005): 1089–91, http://content.nejm.org/cgi/content/full/353/11/1089.

5. American Sleep Apnea Association (www.sleepapnea.org).

6. Cited in Lauren Neergaard, "Snoring? It Could Be Sleep Apnea," Associated Press, FoxNews.com, January 7, 2008, http://www.fox news.com/wires/2008Jan07/0,4670,HealthBeatSleepApnea,00.html.

7. Cited in *The Merck Manual of Medical Information*, 2nd ed. (New York: Simon and Schuster, 2003), 474.

8. Daniel Bates and Claire Ellicott, "Teenager Plunges 25 Ft. After Sleepwalking out of Her Bedroom Window," *Mail Online*, May 20, 2009, http://www.dailymail.co.uk/news/article-1184565/Teenager-plunges-25ft-sleepwalking-bedroom-window—survives-breaking-single-bone.html.

9. Data from National Academy for Childhood Sleep Disorders, cited in Carma Haley, "Taking a Night-Time Stroll," Part 1, "Home and Travel," *iParenting*, http://www.childrentoday.com/resources/articles /sleepwalking.htm (accessed November 19, 2009).

10. Ibid.

11. *Medline Plus Encyclopedia*, s.v. "Nightmares," http://www.nlm.nih .gov/medlineplus/ency/article/003209.htm.

12. Study conducted by Jennifer Parker, University of the West of England, Bristol, cited in "Women 'More Prone to Nightmares,'" *BBC News*, September 11, 2008, http://news.bbc.co.uk/2/hi/7609985.stm (accessed November 19, 2009).

13. Medline Plus Encyclopedia, s.v. "Nightmares."

Chapter 7

1. "The Late Shift," San Gabriel Valley Newspaper Group, March 5, 2007, www.sgvn.com.

2. Cited in Grace Fleming, "Teens and Sleep Deprivation," About.com, "Homework and Study Tips," http://homeworktips.about.com/od /timemanagement/a/sleeptime.htm (accessed November 20, 2009).

3. Study conducted by the Johns Hopkins Bloomberg School of Public Health, published in Xiaoli Chen, May A. Beydoun, and Youfa Wang, "Is Sleep Duration Associated with Childhood Obesity? A Systematic Review and Meta-Analysis," *Obesity* (February 2008); cited in "Reduced Sleep Can Increase Childhood Obesity Risk," *ScienceDaily* (February 8, 2008), http://www.sciencedaily.com/releases /2008/02/080207104303.htm.

4. Elsie M. Taveras et al., "Short Sleep Duration in Infancy and Risk of Childhood Overweight," *Archives of Pediatrics and Adolescent Medicine* 162, no. 4 (April 2008): 305–311, cited in "Infant's Sleep Tied to Childhood Obesity," Newsmax.com, April 8, 2008, http://www .newsmax.com/health/infant_sleep_obesity/2008/04/08/86301.html.

5. Study conducted by Avi Sadeh et al., Tel Aviv University, cited in B. Bower, "Grade-Schoolers Grow into Sleep Loss," *Science News* 157, no. 21 (May 2000): 324, http://www.sciencenews.org/pages/pdfs /data/2000/157-21/15721-04.pdf.

6. National Institutes of Health, National Center on Sleep Disorders Research and Office of Prevention, Education, and Control, *Working Group Report on Problem Sleepiness* (Washington, D.C.: National Institutes of Health, 1997), 1, http://www.nhlbi.nih.gov/health/prof /sleep/pslp_wg.pdf.

7. Jeffrey G. Johnson et al., "Association Between Television Viewing and Sleep Problems During Adolescence and Early Adulthood," *Archives of Pediatrics and Adolescent Medicine* 158, no. 6 (June 2004): 562–68, http://archpedi.ama-assn.org/cgi/content/full/158/6/562

?maxtoshow=&HITS=10&hits=10&RESULTFORMAT=&fulltext =SLEEP&searchid=1&FIRSTINDEX=10&resourcetype=HWCIT.

8. Xianchen Liu, "Sleep and Adolescent Suicidal Behavior," *Journal of Sleep and Sleep Disorders Research* 27, no. 7 (2004): 1351–58, http://psycnet.apa.org/psycinfo/2004-20988-012.

9. Mary A. Carskadon, ed., *Adolescent Sleep Patterns: Biological, Social, and Psychological Influences* (Cambridge, UK: Cambridge University Press, 2004), 4.

10. Dennis Prager, "Excitement Deprives Children of Happiness," Townhall.com, August 7, 2007, http://townhall.com/columnists /dennisprager/2007/08/07/excitement_deprives_children_of _happiness (accessed November 20, 2009).

Chapter 8

1. Studies cited in Tara Parker-Pope, "Marriage Linked with Better Sleep," Health, *New York Times* (June 10, 2009), http://well.blogs.ny times.com/2009/06/10/marriage-linked-with-better-sleep/.

2. Wendy M. Troxel et al., "Attachment Anxiety, Relationship Context, and Sleep in Women with Recurrent Major Depression," *Psychosomatic Medicine* 69 (2007): 692–99, http://www.psychosomatic medicine.org/cgi/content/abstract/69/7/692.

3. National Sleep Foundation, random telephone survey of 1,004 adults, conducted in 2001.

4. Studies cited in American Academy of Pediatrics Policy Statement, "The Changing Concept of Sudden Infant Death Syndrome: Diagnostic Coding Shifts, Controversies Regarding the Sleeping Environment, and New Variables to Consider in Reducing Risk," *Pediatrics* 116, no. 5 (2005), 1248, http://aappolicy.aappublications.org/cgi /reprint/pediatrics;116/5/1245.pdf.

5. Sharon Morris May, *How to Argue So Your Spouse Will Listen* (Nashville: Thomas Nelson, 2007).

Chapter 9

1. National Commission on Sleep Disorders Research, U.S. Department of Health and Human Services, *Wake Up America: A National Sleep Alert, A Report of the National Commission on Sleep Disorders Research* (Washington, D.C.: Government Printing Office, 1993–1995).

2. H. Moldofsky et al., "Effects of Sleep Deprivation on Human Immune Functions," *FASEB Journal* 3 (1989): 1.

3. Archibald D. Hart, *The Anxiety Cure* (Nashville: Thomas Nelson, 2001), 149.

4. Kim Youngsoo et al., "Repeated Sleep Restriction in Rats Leads to Homeostatic and Allostatic Responses During Recovery Sleep," 2007 *Proceedings of the National Academy of Sciences* 104, no. 25, http://www.biomedexperts.com/Abstract.bme/17548824/Repeated _sleep_restriction_in_rats_leads_to_homeostatic_and_allostatic _responses_during_recovery_sleep, cited in Kathleen Fackelmann, "Study: Sleep Deficit May Be Impossible to Make Up," *USA Today*, November 25, 2007, http://www.usatoday.com/news/health /2007-11-25-sleep-deficit_N.htm.

Chapter 10

1. "Americans May Be Relying Too Heavily on Sleeping Pills When Safer Remedies Are Available," Press Room, ConsumerReports.org, September 2006, http://www.consumerreports.org/cro/cu-press-room /pressroom/archive/2006/09/0609_eng0609slp_ov.htm (accessed November 20, 2009).

2. Study cited in "Americans May Be Relying Too Heavily on Sleeping Pills," ConsumerReports.org.

3. Gregg D. Jacobs et al., "Cognitive Behavior Therapy and Pharmacotherapy for Insomnia: A Randomized Controlled Trial and Direct Comparison," *Archives of Internal Medicine* 164, no 17 (September

2004): 1888–96, http://archinte.ama-assn.org/cgi/content/abstract /164/17/1888?ijkey=dd345903f6c5e34b30ee3c199be3b19bebb45b 9e&keytype2=tf_ipsecsha.

4. Data from Medco Health Solutions, cited in Mary Duenwald, "Doctors Ponder Drugs for Sleepless Nights of Adolescence," *New York Times*, November 15, 2005, http://www.nytimes.com/2005/11 /15/health/15cons.html?_r=1&pagewanted=print.

5. Ibid.

6. Ibid

7. Ivy M. Andersen, "Melatonin for Insomnia in Children with Autism Spectrum Disorders," *Journal of Child Neurology* 23, no. 5 (2008): 482–85, http://jcn.sagepub.com/cgi/content/abstract/23/5/482.

Chapter 11

1. Archibald D. Hart, *The Anxiety Cure* (Nashville: Thomas Nelson, 2001).

2. Daniel G. Amen, *Change Your Brain, Change Your Life* (New York: Three Rivers Press, 1999).

Chapter 12

1. John Baillie, "The Theology of Sleep," in *Christian Devotion* (Oxford: Oxford University Press, 1962).

2. Eluned Summers-Bremmer, *Insomnia: A Cultural History* (London: Reaktion Books, 2008), 14.

3. Charles H. Spurgeon, "Refreshing Sleep," in *Faith's Checkbook: A Daily Devotional*, public domain.

4. Archibald D. Hart, *Unlocking the Mystery of Your Emotions* (Waco, TX: Word, 1990).

More Great Resources
from Focus on the Family®

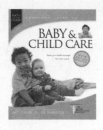

Complete Guide to Baby & Child Care
From Pre-Birth to the Teen Years
Newly revised and expanded with the latest research and medical data, Focus on the Family's ® *Complete Guide to Baby & Child Care* gives you practical knowledge for the privilege of parenting. This comprehensive medical reference book addresses the physical, mental, emotional, and spiritual needs of children.

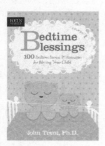

Bedtime Blessings
Make It a Really Good Night!
In *Bedtime Blessings*, you'll find 100 easy-to-follow ideas for terrific tuck-ins, including: read-to-me stories, amazing experiments, intriguing puzzles, "let's pretend" activities, and more! Best of all, each bedtime activity is followed by a prayer. With *Bedtime Blessings*, you'll build a close relationship with your child that can last a lifetime.

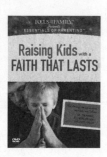

Essentials of Parenting: Raising Kids with
a Faith that Lasts
Hosted by popular counselor and author Dr. Greg Smalley, *Raising Kids with a Faith that Lasts* features top parenting mentors such as Larry Fowler, Mark Holmen, and Dr. Tim Kimmel. Topics include: introducing your child to faith, creating a faith plan for your family, assessing the spiritual needs of your children, and practical tips for day-to-day life. The six lessons on this DVD will provide inspiration and insight to help parents raise kids with a *faith that lasts*.

FOR MORE INFORMATION

 Online:
Log on to FocusOnTheFamily.com
In Canada, log on to focusonthefamily.ca.

 Phone:
Call toll free: 800-A-FAMILY
In Canada, call toll free: 800-661-9800.

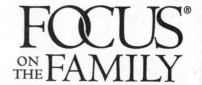

BPZZXP1